EMERGENCY
TELEPHONE NUMBERS

Doctor _____

Doctor _____

Doctor _____

Ambulance

    (911, 0, or local emergency number) _____

Police department _____

Fire department _____

Local poison control center _____

Hospital emergency department _____

Health insurance emergency

    preapproval number _____

Work numbers _____

_____

Dentist _____

Baby-sitter _____

Neighborhood pharmacy _____

24-hour pharmacy _____

Electric company _____

Gas company _____

Neighbors _____

_____

_____

Relative _____

Local board of health _____

IMMEDIATE TREATMENT

- Call out for someone to get help.
- Look, listen, and feel for breathing (see p. 36).
- Determine if the victim's heart is beating (see CPR, p. 36).
- Stop excessive bleeding (see p. 96).
- If something has been swallowed, ask victim what it was.
- Treat for shock (see p. 240).
- Perform the Heimlich maneuver for choking (see p. 51).

WHAT TO TELL THE DOCTOR OR PARAMEDICS

- What has happened.
- The victim's noticeable injuries, symptoms, or signs.
- When the accident occurred or the symptoms or signs began.
- What medications the victim has taken (if known).
- If poisoning has occurred, what has been swallowed, how much, and when.
- Where you and/or the victim are.
- The phone number of your location.

WHAT TO TELL THE POISON CONTROL CENTER

- The poisoning victim's name, phone number, age, and approximate weight.
- The exact name of the ingested product and its ingredients and manufacturer (have the container or label at hand when you make the call).
- How much of the product was swallowed.
- When the poisoning occurred or symptoms began.
- The victim's symptoms.
- What first aid, if any, has been performed.
- Medical history of the victim and any current medications he or she is taking.

Compliments of

Aurora Medical Center

Aurora Medical Center	(920) 456-6000
Emergency Department	(920) 456-7400
Walk-In Care	(920) 303-8700

855 N. Westhaven Drive
Oshkosh, WI 54904

www.AuroraHealthCare.org

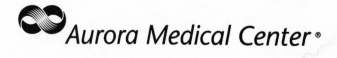

American
Medical
Association

HANDBOOK OF FIRST AID AND EMERGENCY CARE

R E V I S E D   E D I T I O N

Jerrold B. Leikin, MD
Medical Editor,
Emergency Medicine

Bernard J. Feldman, MD
Medical Editor,
Sports Medicine

Stanley M. Zydlo, Jr, MD,
James A. Hill, MD
Medical Editors,
Previous Edition

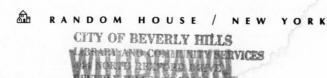

RANDOM HOUSE / NEW YORK

Copyright © 1980, 1990, 2000 by American Medical Association

All rights reserved under International and Pan-American Copyright Conventions. Published in the United States by Random House, an imprint of The Random House Publishing Group, a division of Random House, Inc., New York, and simultaneously in Canada by Random House of Canada Limited, Toronto.

RANDOM HOUSE and colophon are registered trademarks of Random House, Inc.

Earlier editions of this work were published in 1980 and 1990 by Random House, Inc.

Library of Congress Cataloging-in-Publication Data

American Medical Association handbook of first aid and emergency
  care /developed by the American Medical Association; medical editors,
  Stanley M. Zydlo, Jr., James A. Hill.—Rev. ed.
     p. cm.
   ISBN 0-375-75486-5 (alk. paper)
   1. First aid in illness and injury—Handbooks, manuals, etc.
I. Zydlo, Stanley M. II. Hill, James A., 1950– . III. American
Medical Association. IV. Title: Handbook of first aid
and emergency care.
RC86.8.A426 1999
616.02'52—dc21   99-14152

Random House website address: www.atrandom.com

Printed in the United States of America

9 8

Second Revised Edition

Book design by Jo Anne Metsch

FOREWORD

If a medical emergency were to strike you or a member of your family, would you be prepared to handle it? If a stranger collapsed in front of you, could you provide the necessary care at a moment's notice?

Of course, we hope that you never have to face an emergency situation. But when serious illness or injury does occur, providing first aid within the critical first few minutes can save a life. And when you perform first aid correctly, paramedics and doctors can provide their care more effectively.

When you have to deal with more minor occurrences—washing a scraped elbow or knee, or stopping a nosebleed—you will feel better knowing that you are handling the situation in the best way. And you will be better able to offer that all-important reassuring, kind word to the person who is hurt or sick.

Our purpose in publishing this revised edition of the *American Medical Association Handbook of First Aid and Emergency Care* is to help prepare you and your family for both major or minor emergencies. We hope that you take the time now to read through the procedures in this new edition, so that you are familiar with the new information. Please bear in mind that a book cannot take the place of formal training in lifesaving procedures such as cardiopulmonary resuscitation or rescue breathing. We strongly encourage you to take a class from the American Red Cross, the American Heart Association, or your local hospital or fire department.

The American Medical Association wishes you and your family healthy, safe lives.

E. Ratcliffe Anderson, Jr, MD
Executive Vice President
Chief Executive Officer
American Medical Association

JERROLD B. LEIKIN, MD, is the Associate Director of the Emergency Department and is a Senior Attending Physician at Rush-Presbyterian-St. Luke's Medical Center in Chicago. He is also Associate Director of the Toxicon Consortium and holds an appointment as Professor of Medicine at Rush Medical College.

BERNARD J. FELDMAN, MD, practices orthopedics and sports medicine at Great Lakes Orthopedics in Berwyn, Illinois. He is a National Team Physician for the US Greco-Roman Wrestling team, and has been a team physician with the Chicago White Sox since 1982. Dr. Feldman also teaches in the Emergency Services Department at Rush-Presbyterian-St. Luke's Medical Center in Chicago.

ACKNOWLEDGMENTS

Dianna W. Bolen, MA, LCPC

Anthony Burda, RPH

Jack Clifton, MD

Paul K. Harashiro, MD

Karen Judy, MD

Jane Kramer, MD

Karen Newton, RN

Laurie A. Peschke, MSW, LCSW

Michelle Ryan Bartlett

CONTENTS

HOW TO USE THIS BOOK

In serious emergencies, first-aid treatment in the first few minutes can save a life. If you know what to do and act quickly and calmly before medical help arrives, you will enable medical personnel to provide the most effective treatment possible when they get to the scene. In less serious situations, when injury or illness is minor, knowing what to do can save needless visits to the doctor.

This book is designed to meet your immediate needs in emergency situations. To help you find the information you need quickly and easily, the book is divided into three parts.

READ NOW

Part I, Being Prepared for Injuries and Emergencies, contains general information that you should read *now,* so that you will be better prepared to handle an emergency if it occurs.

Part I has seven sections:

• Planning for an Emergency—Now
• Safeguarding Your Home Against Accidents
• When to Call a Doctor
• Ambulance Services and Hospital Emergency Departments
• Recognizing Medical Problems
• First-Aid Techniques to Learn and Practice
• Emergency Procedures to Know

WHEN AN EMERGENCY OCCURS

Part II, Alphabetical Listing of Injuries and Illnesses, is arranged for quick access at the time of an emergency. Injuries and illnesses are listed in alphabetical order, and each entry contains step-by-step treatment for specific problems.

If you have trouble finding the entry you need, a comprehensive index at the back of the book helps you find the appropriate entry.

QUICK REFERENCE: SPORTS FIRST AID

Part III, Sports First Aid, is a fully illustrated listing of the most common sports injuries, arranged by the part of the body that has been injured. Each entry contains information about immediate treatment of the injury, as well as a description of the medical care you may require.

PART I

BEING PREPARED FOR INJURIES AND EMERGENCIES

PLANNING FOR
AN EMERGENCY—NOW

MEDICAL CHART

One of the first things you should do is fill in, for each family member, the medical chart provided at the end of this book. The chart provides medical information you and doctors or paramedics need in an emergency, such as allergies, medications taken regularly, or chronic conditions. There is also a place for important emergency telephone numbers in the front of the book. *Fill these out now,* before you forget.

KNOW THE ROUTE TO THE HOSPITAL

Know the best route to the nearest hospital emergency department. If an ambulance or paramedic team is not available, you may have to drive yourself or a victim to the hospital. It is a good idea to make a practice run so that the roads will be familiar to you at the time of an emergency. Wrong turns can take precious minutes and could mean the difference between life and death.

EMERGENCY MEDICAL IDENTIFICATION

Wearing an emergency ID bracelet or necklace or carrying an emergency information card could save the life of someone who is unable to speak after a serious accident. This medical identification is particularly important for a person who has a chronic condition such as diabetes, epilepsy, glaucoma, or hemophilia, or who may have a serious allergic reaction to certain medications (such as penicillin) or to insect stings.

These bracelets, necklaces, and cards include such information as the individual's name, address, blood type, and any serious conditions or allergies. They should be worn or carried at all times. A bracelet or necklace is generally better than a card since it is more easily noticed. These items are available through several manufacturers. Ask your doctor, hospital emergency department, or local medical association where you might order them.

In the meantime, you can make your own ID card. Include your name, address, telephone number, name and telephone number of a relative to contact, your doctor's name and number, any serious medical conditions or surgical procedures, medication taken regularly, allergies, and any other important information. Be sure the card is prominently displayed in your wallet.

ORGAN DONATION

The need for donated organs far exceeds the supply. For every person who receives an organ transplant each year, many more who could benefit from a transplanted organ will not have the opportunity and will die as a result. If you want to donate your organs after your death, make your intentions clear to your relatives and sign a donor card. Anyone can donate his or her organs and tissues. A person under 18 who wishes to become an organ donor must have his or her parent or legal guardian witness the signing of the donor card. (Parents should keep a copy of their child's donor card in their wallet with their own card.) You should know, however, that even if a person has signed a donor card, some states require the consent of a close relative (parent or legal guardian, spouse, adult child, or adult sibling) before the organs can be donated upon death. For this reason, it is especially important to make your wishes clear to your family.

You can obtain information or applications by calling the Coalition on Donation (800-355-SHARE) or visiting the federal government–sponsored web site (http://www.organdonor.gov). You can also indicate your wish to be an organ donor on your driver's license; ask the secretary of state's office how to do so.

SUPPLIES TO KEEP ON HAND

Now is the time to assemble those basic items you may need when an injury or illness occurs in your home, car, or boat, or while camping. Keep these items together in a box or other container and out of the sight and reach of young children. Be sure to check the supplies periodically and replace used items. If a member of your family has special needs, ask your doctor what additional items you should include.

Keep on hand:

- Different sizes of sterile adhesive strips
- Roll of gauze bandage (3 inches wide)
- Nonstick sterile gauze pads (4 inches × 4 inches) packaged separately in sealed wrappers
- Butterfly bandages and thin adhesive strips to hold skin edges together
- Roll of adhesive tape (1 inch wide)
- Scissors
- Elastic bandage (2 or 3 inches wide) for wrapping sprained ankles and wrists
- Package of cotton-tipped swabs
- Roll of absorbent cotton to pad a splint
- Acetaminophen, ibuprofen, or naproxen for pain relief (in liquid or tablet form for children)
- Thermometers
- Small jar or tube of petroleum jelly to use with rectal thermometer
- 1-ounce bottle of syrup of ipecac to induce vomiting if poisons are swallowed; activated charcoal solution to prevent the stomach from absorbing poison
- Tweezers without teeth
- Safety pins
- Small bottle of 3 percent hydrogen peroxide
- Tube of 1 percent hydrocortisone cream
- Bar of plain soap
- Flashlight for car or boat, or when camping
- Antihistamine such as diphenhydramine in liquid or tablet form for allergic reactions
- Bottle of povidone-iodine solution
- Bottle of sterile saline solution or irrigation fluid to wash out eyes
- Sunscreen with a sun protection factor (SPF) of at least 15
- Tooth preservation kit

EVERYDAY ITEMS THAT CAN BE USED IN AN EMERGENCY

Certain everyday items in your home can be used in an emergency (keep in mind other items that may also be useful under urgent circumstances):

- Disposable or regular diapers, sanitary napkins, towels, sheets, or linens to use as compresses to control heavy bleeding, for bandages, as padding for splints, or in emergency childbirth
- Diaper pins to secure bandage or sling
- Blankets to keep the victim warm
- Magazines, newspapers, umbrella, or pillow to use as splints for broken bones
- Table leaf or old door to use as a stretcher
- Fan and/or a spray bottle of water to cool heatstroke victim
- Large scarf or handkerchief to use as eye bandage or sling

SAFEGUARDING YOUR HOME
AGAINST ACCIDENTS

Keeping your home safe for you and your family should be your #1 health priority. Accidents, including those that occur in the home, are a major cause of death in the United States. Most of these deaths could have been prevented.

To ensure that your home is safe, take a few minutes to read over the items listed below, and review them annually. The list is by no means all-inclusive. Other areas of the home to check regularly for safety hazards include closets, the attic, and additional storage areas such as garden sheds.

One last reminder: Smoke detectors, carbon monoxide detectors, and fire extinguishers are necessary investments that can save lives. Check them each month to ensure they are in working order. Change the batteries every year on an easy-to-remember day such as your birthday.

KITCHEN

- Chemical cleaners: Tightly cap or close and properly store (in their original container and with a label) out of the sight and reach of children and away from food. Never reuse containers for storing food or other items.
- Liquor: Properly store out of the sight and reach of children.
- Knives: Properly store out of the sight and reach of children.
- Throw rugs: Tack down, hold in place with carpet tape, or remove.
- Cords on electrical appliances: Fix or replace if frayed.
- Oven and stove top: Clean regularly.
- Refrigerator and freezer: Clean and defrost regularly.
- Microwave oven: Clean regularly and properly house on a countertop or cart.
- Other electrical appliances: Clean and properly store.
- Medications: Store in a locked cabinet and discard expired medicines by flushing down the toilet. Keep track of medications by writing them down in the chart on p. 338.

BATHROOM

- Glass containers: Remove or replace with plastic containers.
- Chemical cleaners: Tightly cap or close and properly store out of the sight and reach of children.
- Hair dryer, curling iron, electric shaver: Unplug and properly store.
- Rugs or mats: Tack down, hold in place with carpet tape, or remove.
- Tub and shower: Place adhesive grippers on floor of tub and install railing along wall to help prevent falls.
- Medications (see Kitchen).

LIVING ROOM

- Walls and windowsills: Remove peeling paint.
- Plants: Remove any poisonous plants.
- Ashtrays: Discard cigarette butts and keep matches and lighters out of the sight and reach of children.
- Fireplace: Screen off fireplace.

STAIRS

- Handrails: Extend the full length of the stairs at least on one side.
- Rugs or mats: Remove from top and bottom of stairs.
- Lighting: Adequately illuminate all steps.

GARAGE OR BASEMENT

- Cleaners and chemicals such as rat poison, weed killer, antifreeze, paint, paint thinner, or charcoal lighter fluid: Tightly cap or close and properly store out of the sight and reach of children. Never reuse an empty container to store other items. Throw out old paint. Immediately clean up spills.
- Gasoline can: Tightly close and properly store out of the sight and reach of children. Immediately clean up spills.
- Saws, chisels, or other items with sharp blades: Properly store out of the sight and reach of children.
- Electric tools: Keep unplugged and with safety locks on.
- Old rags or newspapers: Discard.

- Loose cords or hoses: Properly roll up and store.
- Doors, windows, and screens: Properly store.
- Lighting: Adequately illuminate all areas, including corners.
- Buckets: Empty and properly store. Infants and young children can drown in fluid-filled buckets.

CAR

- Seat belts: Wear a lap and shoulder seat belt whenever you drive or ride in a car, and make sure all passengers in your car wear theirs.
- Child safety seats: Keep a child who weighs less than 60 pounds in a safety seat appropriate to his or her age and weight at all times. Make sure that a child over 60 pounds always wears a lap and shoulder belt. Never allow a child under 12 to sit in the front seat of a car that has a front passenger seat air bag.
- Drugs: Never drive after drinking alcohol or taking other drugs that could impair your judgment or concentration.
- Maintenance: Keep your car in good repair, especially the lights, brakes, and tires.

SWIMMING POOL

- Signs and markings: Clearly mark depths on the deck near the edge and along the sides of the pool. Place or paint "NO DIVING" signs on the deck near the shallow end.
- Floats and safety devices: Place floats across the width of the pool to mark where the deep end starts. Provide approved floating safety devices and ensure that they are not removed.
- Rules: Never allow running on the deck. Never allow diving in an above-ground pool. Allow diving in an in-ground pool only if the water is more than 9 feet deep and there is sufficient distance between the diving board and the slope up to the shallow end.

WHEN TO CALL A DOCTOR

At some time you may need to call a doctor about an injury or other medical problem. If the problem is a real emergency such as severe bleeding, a possible heart attack or stroke, a diabetic coma, or severe abdominal pain, call paramedics or an ambulance service to take the victim to the hospital.

If you are unsure of the victim's condition and he or she has severe or prolonged symptoms such as pain, vomiting and/or diarrhea (particularly with blood), difficulty breathing, or high fever, call a doctor—regardless of the hour.

It is very helpful when calling the doctor to give him or her specific information regarding the victim. Be prepared to tell the doctor or nurse the following:

- What has happened.
- The victim's noticeable injuries, symptoms, or signs.
- When the accident occurred or the symptoms or signs began.
- What medications the victim has taken (if known).
- If poisoning has occurred, what has been swallowed, how much, and when.
- Where you and/or the victim are.
- The phone number of your location.

Above all else—and especially in an emergency situation—try to remain calm and follow the doctor's or medical professional's instructions. Ask what more you can do to help. Your first-aid measures could save valuable seconds and, possibly, the life of the victim.

AMBULANCE SERVICES AND HOSPITAL EMERGENCY DEPARTMENTS

In an emergency, time is critical. For emergencies that appear serious or life-threatening, call 911 (or your local emergency number), 0 for operator, or an ambulance service and ask for immediate transportation to a hospital emergency department. It is necessary to call an ambulance to take an injured or ill person to a hospital emergency department anytime his or her symptoms are critical or life-threatening, such as in cases of severe head, neck, or back injury; drug overdose; severe allergic reaction; or unconsciousness. In these instances, the victim should be transported to the hospital as quickly as possible. If an ambulance is late or unavailable, *you* may have to drive the victim to the hospital.

AMBULANCE SERVICES AND PARAMEDICS

Most communities have some type of ambulance service and specialized emergency medical personnel available. The most highly trained personnel are emergency medical technician (EMT) paramedics. They are trained to administer advanced life-support techniques such as cardiopulmonary resuscitation (CPR), to take electrocardiographic (ECG) tracings that reveal the electrical activity of the heart, to start intravenous (IV) lines, and to give medication.

Other trained medical personnel can provide CPR and perform emergency medical procedures, such as splinting broken bones. Some can shock a victim's heart with specialized equipment if the heart has stopped beating. They cannot, however, administer medication or perform sophisticated medical procedures.

Many ambulances with paramedics have telemetry equipment hooked up to a local hospital to relay the ECG readings to hospital physicians. A doctor's instructions can then be relayed back to the paramedics via radio.

11

If you have children, you should know that not all hospital emergency departments have personnel trained to handle childhood emergencies or equipment designed to treat children. Call the emergency departments at the hospitals nearest your home and ask if they are equipped to handle pediatric emergencies. If you find a children's emergency department or an emergency department that is equipped to handle pediatric emergencies, keep the number near your phone so that you can call there for help in an emergency. Make sure you know the exact location in case you need to drive your child there.

Your community may have an ambulance service that provides transportation to the hospital but offers little or no emergency care. The attendants of such vehicles may not be trained to provide care beyond performing simple first aid.

Paramedics and other ambulance personnel are usually available through various community resources such as the fire department, police department, volunteer associations, and funeral homes. Check with the resources in your community before an emergency strikes so that you will know the type of service to call. Paramedics should not be called for minor illnesses or injuries such as sprained ankles, minor cuts, or colds; they need to be available to treat people who have more serious conditions. Often victims with minor injuries can be driven to the hospital by a family member or friend.

WHEN TO GO TO THE EMERGENCY DEPARTMENT

Anytime the victim's symptoms *appear* critical or life-threatening, or anytime someone is experiencing severe pain, he or she must be taken to the hospital. Any situation that *seems* like an emergency warrants a trip to a hospital emergency department. If you have time and the person's health insurance plan recommends preapproval for emergency department visits, call for approval. But don't take the time to call if the situation is critical. Most plans cover emergency department visits, even without preapproval, and it's much more important to get the victim timely medical care. It's also a good idea to contact the person's doctor.

If you are taking someone to the hospital and there is time, call ahead to the emergency department or have someone else call. Tell them you are coming, the nature of the victim's injury or illness, and the name and phone number of the victim's doctor. This enables the staff to know what to expect, to prepare for the victim's arrival, and to contact his or her doctor.

When the victim arrives at the hospital, he or she may have to wait if the emergency department is busy, unless his or her condition is serious or critical.

INFORMATION TO GIVE EMERGENCY DEPARTMENT PERSONNEL

Emergency department personnel treat the most serious and critical cases first. Any specific information you can give them about the victim's condition will help them determine its seriousness. Describing specific complaints, such as severe crushing chest pain or sharp lower abdominal pain, is very helpful. Other useful information includes:

- When the symptoms began.
- What makes the pain or condition better or worse and whether the pain has traveled to another part of the body.
- What the victim was doing when the injury or illness occurred.
- What changes have occurred in the victim since the onset of the illness or injury.
- What the victim has swallowed, if anything.
- What medications the victim has been taking.

If time allows before leaving for the hospital, gather insurance identification cards, Medicare or Medicaid cards, or any other record of medical benefits to which the victim is entitled. Be prepared to give the victim's name, age, address, a history of major injuries or illnesses, and known allergies.

Laboratory tests and x-rays may be necessary to help make a diagnosis while initial treatment is being given. Depending upon the size and the location of the hospital, most emergency departments offer full medical services, ranging from bandaging a cut to surgery. If the emergency department cannot handle a specific situation, it must arrange to send the victim to another hospital that is capable of handling the medical problem.

Emergency department treatment is generally more expensive than medical treatment received in a doctor's office. Most emergency departments must be staffed with doctors, nurses, and other personnel on a 24-hour basis, thus increasing their costs. Also, emergency departments must be equipped with costly equipment not usually found in a doctor's office. Most hospitals will process insurance forms. A number of hospitals are now also accepting major credit cards for payment.

Fever, an unusually slow or fast pulse, and changes in the size of the pupils are common signs of possible health problems. Temperature and pulse rates have different meanings for children and adults. Knowing how to take a temperature, find a pulse, and recognize changes in the eyes can help you evaluate a potential problem and provide important information to doctors.

TAKING A TEMPERATURE

Several different types of thermometers are available. Digital thermometers are easy to use and record a temperature quickly (in less than 30 seconds) and accurately. Glass thermometers are the least expensive, but they take 3 to 4 minutes to record a temperature and can be difficult to read. Tympanic (ear) thermometers, which measure the amount of infrared radiation in the eardrum, are not as accurate in infants under age 1 year, so doctors don't recommend them for children this age. Ear thermometers are, however, accurate and convenient for older children and adults.

Most temperatures are taken by mouth with an oral (Fahrenheit or Celsius) thermometer. People with mouth injuries should have their temperature taken with an ear thermometer, and children under 3 years should have their temperature taken rectally with a rectal thermometer.

The average normal temperature taken by mouth is 98.6° Fahrenheit, plus or minus 1°. A Celsius thermometer, common in Canada and Europe, may be used instead of a Fahrenheit thermometer. An average normal temperature on a Celsius thermometer is 37°, plus or minus 1°.

An infant's temperature, taken rectally (with a rectal Fahrenheit or Celsius thermometer), usually registers 1° higher than a normal oral temperature. (A temperature taken by mouth registers lower than a temperature taken rectally because air entering the mouth cools the mouth slightly, thus lowering the temperature *reading*.)

How to Read a Thermometer

Digital thermometers and ear thermometers are easy to read because they display the temperature reading on a small screen. To read a glass thermometer, hold the end without the bulb between the thumb and the first finger. Use good light. Look through the pointed edge toward the flat side until you see a thin silver or red line coming out of the bulb. Rotate the thermometer slightly if the silver line is not visible. The temperature reading is at the end of the silver line. The long lines mark the degrees of temperature and the short lines indicate two tenths of a degree. An arrow points to the normal reading of 98.6°F (37°C). Readings higher than this indicate a fever, except in a rectal temperature, which is normally 1° higher.

Before taking a temperature with a glass thermometer, you need to shake the thermometer until the silver or red line reads below the 98.6°F (37°C) mark to approximately 95°F (35°C). Hold the thermometer as described above and shake it sharply downward with a snapping wrist movement. Read the thermometer to make sure the mercury is shaken down.

How to Take an Oral Temperature

If you are using an oral thermometer, insert the bulb under the tongue. Keep the thermometer in place for 2 to 3 minutes if you are using a glass thermometer or 30 seconds or until you hear the beep for a digital thermometer. Warn the person not to talk or bite on the thermometer. *Do not* take a temperature for at least 10 minutes after a person has taken a bath, smoked, eaten hot or cold foods, or drunk water; this can affect the temperature reading.

If you have trouble reading the glass thermometer, set it aside until someone else can read it. The temperature reading on a glass thermometer will stay the same until the thermometer is shaken down. The temperature display on a digital thermometer lasts about 3 minutes.

How to Take a Rectal Temperature

To take a rectal temperature, place the infant or young child on his or her stomach on a firm surface or on your lap. Lubricate the bulb end of the thermometer with petroleum jelly, separate the cheeks of the child's buttocks so that the rectum is visible, and gently insert the thermometer into the rectum about ¹/₂ to 1 inch. Never use force. If you meet resistance, change the direction of the thermometer slightly. Hold the thermometer firmly between your fingers and squeeze the child's buttocks together with your other hand. Leave the thermometer in place for about 30 seconds or until you hear the beep for a digital thermometer, or 2 to 3 minutes for a glass thermometer. If the child struggles, hold him or her steady by placing your hand on the small of his or her back.

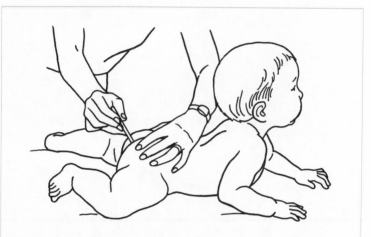

TAKING A RECTAL TEMPERATURE

To take an infant's or young child's temperature rectally, place the child on his or her stomach on a firm surface (or on your lap). Separate the cheeks of the child's buttocks and gently insert the thermometer into the rectum about ½ to 1 inch. Hold the thermometer firmly between your fingers and squeeze the child's buttocks together with your other hand.

FINDING A PULSE RATE

The normal pulse rate for an adult at rest can range from 60 to 100 beats per minute. Well-conditioned athletes may have markedly lower pulse rates (50 to 60 beats per minute). Rates also can vary if you are excited or have just completed exercise or any other activity. To find your normal resting pulse rate, place three fingertips of one hand at your wrist just below the thumb on the palm side of your other hand. Count the pulsations for 60 seconds. Or, count for 15 seconds and multiply by 4. This is your pulse rate. Be sure to do this when you are rested and quiet, not after activity or emotional excitement.

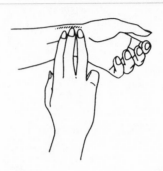

HOW TO FIND A PULSE
To find a pulse, place three fingertips at the wrist just below the thumb.

Pulse rates in children vary according to age. The average pulse rate for a newborn infant is about 120 beats per minute. To find the pulse rate in infants, check below the left nipple or on the brachial artery, located on the inside of the arm between the elbow and the shoulder. Pulse rate in a child 1 to 5 years old can be anywhere between 90 and 120 beats per minute. A child 5 to 15 years old has a pulse rate between 70 and 100.

A resting pulse rate that is higher or lower than a person's usual rate can indicate a medical emergency. If your resting pulse rate or that of a family member is significantly higher or lower than usual, call 911 (or your local emergency number) or go immediately to the nearest hospital emergency department.

RECOGNIZING CHANGES IN THE PUPILS

Pupils are the dark, central portions of the eyes. Dilated (very large) or constricted (very small) pupils can indicate a medical problem. To recognize these conditions in yourself or someone else, you first need to know how normal pupils look. The best way to do this is to look at your own eyes in a mirror. Normal

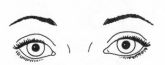

Normal pupils are fairly small.

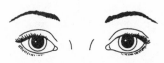

Dilated pupils are large and cover a large area of the irides.

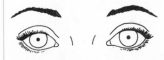

Constricted pupils can be very small, about 1/16 of an inch in diameter.

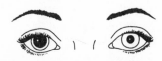

Pupils that are unequal in size may indicate a serious medical condition that requires prompt medical attention.

CHECKING THE PUPILS

The pupil is located in the center of the iris (the colored part of the eye). A change in the pupils can indicate a medical problem.

pupils are fairly small. Dilated pupils are quite large. Constricted pupils are like pinpoints, about 1/16 of an inch in diameter.

Pupils that are noticeably different in size from one another can indicate a serious medical problem and may occur from a head injury, a stroke, or a previous eye injury. If you notice pupils that are unequal in size in yourself or in another person, seek prompt medical attention at a physician's office or hospital emergency department. (See Head, Neck, and Back Injuries, p. 194, and Stroke, p. 250.)

COMMON MEDICAL SYMPTOMS

There are several symptoms that all of us experience from time to time. The most common are fever, nausea, and headache. These symptoms may or may not indicate a serious medical condition.

Fever most often indicates that an infection is present. A fever also may occur with asthma or allergies. In some cases, chills may precede a fever. A fever over 105°F (40.6°C) always requires medical attention. (See Asthma, p. 70; Chills, p. 136; Breathing Problems in Children [Croup], p. 103; Fever, p. 180; and Headaches, p. 203.)

Nausea is a sick feeling in the stomach and is often accompanied by a desire to vomit. Nausea can be an early sign of pregnancy or a symptom of problems such as excessive eating or drinking, allergic reactions to insect stings or spider or snake bites, drug withdrawal, reactions to medications, motion sickness, heart attack, heat exhaustion, food poisoning, fainting, vertigo, infections, appendicitis, and bowel obstruction. (See information about these conditions in Part II.)

Headaches are most commonly caused by muscle tightening under the scalp, often the result of emotional tension. Other causes of headaches include infections, allergies, high blood pressure, multiple insect stings, head injuries, heat exhaustion, food poisoning, stroke, and brain tumors. They can also be danger signals in pregnancy. (See entries for these conditions in Part II.)

If a headache is accompanied by other symptoms, such as nausea, fever, vomiting, a stiff neck, or visual disturbances (such as loss of vision, double vision, or blurred vision), seek immediate medical attention. (See Headaches, p. 203.)

ALARMING MEDICAL SYMPTOMS

Certain symptoms, such as seizures, can be more frightening to experience or watch than they are medically dangerous. This does not mean, however, that you should ignore these conditions. All severe or prolonged symptoms should be reported to your doctor.

Certain other symptoms, such as the sudden onset of chest pain or the sudden loss of vision in one eye, indicate serious medical conditions. In such cases, the victim should be transported without delay to a physician's office or to a hospital emergency department. At all times, try to remain calm so that your reaction does not frighten the victim.

Seizures in children are most commonly caused by a rapid rise in temperature due to an acute infection. These seizures (called febrile seizures) seldom last longer than 2 to 3 minutes. (If these seizures—also called convulsions—last longer, seek immediate medical treatment at a hospital emergency department.) All febrile seizures should be reported to your doctor.

Epileptic seizures are another common type of seizure, which usually occur in people who have a hereditary tendency to have seizures. However, epileptic seizures may occur when some brain cells temporarily become overactive and release too much electrical energy, stimulating part or all of the brain. The primary aim is to prevent the person from harming himself or herself. Contrary to myth, a person having a seizure is not in danger of biting off or swallowing his or her tongue. Do *not* put any object into the person's mouth. After the seizure is over, consult a doctor. (See Seizures, p. 237.)

Severe headache that comes on suddenly with fever, nausea, vomiting, or visual disturbances, or in conjunction with a stiff neck, requires immediate medical attention. A severe headache of this kind may be symptomatic of meningitis, encephalitis, stroke, or a tumor. (See Headaches, p. 203.)

Loss of consciousness that occurs suddenly and without warning may indicate a stroke or a heart attack, or that a person has stopped breathing. He or she may require cardiopulmonary resuscitation (CPR). Refer to information about CPR on pp. 30–50. (See also Unconsciousness, p. 259.)

Severe chest pain or tightness (especially if accompanied by sweating) that occurs suddenly and without warning may signal a heart attack and is a life-threatening emergency. (See Heart Attack, p. 204.)

Loss of vision in one eye or numbness or weakness on one side of the body that occurs suddenly and without warning may be the onset of a stroke. Seek medical attention immediately. (See Stroke, p. 250.)

Sudden loss of sensation or motion in an arm or leg may result from a stroke or a brain tumor. The condition should be brought to the attention of a physician without delay. Do not wait until the symptom goes away. Even if the symptom *does* disappear, seek medical attention. (See Stroke, p. 250.)

Shortness of breath for no apparent reason may mean the onset of an asthma attack or an acute allergic reaction, or may be symptomatic of congestive heart failure. Seek medical attention immediately to rule out a serious medical condition. (See also Asthma, p. 70.)

Blood in the urine may signal an infection, kidney stone, or malignancy.

Blood in the stool or blood in vomit may signal an ulcer or bowel or stomach cancer. These symptoms require immediate medical attention.

FIRST-AID TECHNIQUES TO LEARN AND PRACTICE

Dressings, bandages, slings, and splints are an important part of first-aid care. It is a good idea to learn and practice their application before an emergency strikes. Knowing how to apply a dressing, bandage, or splint will enable you to do so calmly and expertly during a stressful situation.

DRESSINGS

A dressing, or compress, is a covering placed directly over a wound. Its purpose is to help control bleeding, absorb secretions from the wound, and prevent contamination by germs. Because the dressing is placed directly over the wound, it should be sterile. Sterile dressings such as gauze pads and bandages are individually wrapped and are available at most drugstores. If a sterile dressing is not available, a clean handkerchief, pillowcase, sheet, or other cloth can be used. If time allows, a cloth boiled in water for 15 minutes and then dried will provide a sterile dressing. Adhesive tape and fluffy materials such as absorbent cotton should never be applied directly to the wound, as they can stick to the wound and be difficult to remove.

The dressing should be large enough to cover an area 1 inch beyond all edges of the wound, to prevent contamination of any part of the wound. To apply the dressing, hold it directly over the wound and lower it into place. *Do not* slide or drag the dressing over the skin, as this contaminates the dressing. Discard any dressing that has slipped out of place before it has been bandaged.

BANDAGES

A bandage is a piece of material that holds a dressing or splint in place. It can also be a wrap, such as an elastic bandage, that is applied directly to an injured area to help decrease bleeding or swelling or lend support to a joint or group of muscles. Most bandages can be purchased at drugstores.

To function properly, a bandage must be applied snugly *but not too tightly*. A bandage applied too tightly can cut off circulation and cause serious tissue damage. An elastic bandage, though very effective if applied properly, can be particularly dangerous because of the tendency to stretch it too tightly. Remember that an injured area may swell, causing a snug bandage to become too tight.

When applying a bandage to the arm, hand, leg, or foot, leave the fingertips or toes exposed so that danger signals such as swelling, bluish or pale color, or coldness can be observed or felt. If any of these signs appear or if the victim complains of numbness or tingling, loosen the bandage immediately.

Common Adhesive Bandages

Rectangular Bandages
A rectangular bandage is used for simple cuts and scrapes and can be purchased at most drugstores. The rectangular bandage is a combination of both dressing and bandage. To prevent contamination, do not touch the gauze dressing while applying it to the wound.

Butterfly Bandages and Narrow Adhesive Strips
Butterfly bandages and narrow adhesive strips are thin pieces of tape that are used to hold the edges of a cut together, thus allowing the wound to heal. They are especially useful in treating small cuts. When applying the bandage, gently hold the edges of the cut together.

COMMON ADHESIVE BANDAGES
A rectangular bandage (*left*), a combination of both dressing and bandage, is used for simple cuts and scrapes. The butterfly bandage (*center*) and the narrow adhesive strip (*right*) are thin pieces of tape that are used to hold the edges of a cut together.

Roller Gauze Bandages

The roller bandage comes in various widths and lengths and is usually made of gauze. It comes packaged in rolls and can be used on most parts of the body. If commercial roller bandages are not available, a bandage can be made from a clean strip of cloth. The most common uses of roller gauze are for circular, figure-of-eight, and fingertip bandages.

Circular Bandages

A circular bandage is the easiest to apply. It is used on areas that do not vary much in width, such as the wrist, toes, and fingers. To apply a circular bandage:

1. Anchor the bandage by placing the end of it at a slight angle over the affected part and making several circular turns to hold the end in place. Don't wrap the bandage too tightly.

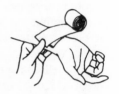

2. Make additional circular turns by overlapping the preceding strip by approximately ¾ of its width. Continue circling the bandage in the same direction until the dressing is completely covered.

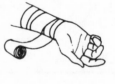

3. To secure the bandage, cut the gauze with scissors or a knife and apply adhesive tape or a safety pin to the bandage. Or tie a loop knot by extending the rolled gauze out about 8 inches away from the part being bandaged. Place your thumb or two fingers in the middle of the rolled-out gauze and pull that section of the gauze (from the fingers to the gauze roll) in the same direction as you did in applying the bandage. The remainder of the gauze and roll will be on the opposite side. If scissors are available, cut the gauze.

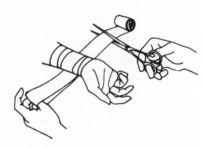

25

4. Check that the doubled gauze is on one side and the single gauze is on the other.
5. Tie a knot over the bandage.

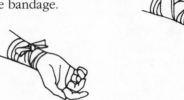

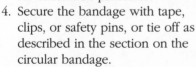

Figure-of-Eight Bandages

A figure-of-eight bandage is particularly useful for the ankle, wrist, and hand. To apply a figure-of-eight bandage:

1. Anchor the bandage with one or two circular turns around the affected part, being careful not to wrap the bandage too tightly.

2. To make the figure-of-eight, bring the bandage diagonally across the top of the foot, around the ankle, down across the top of the foot, and under the arch.

3. Continue these figure-of-eight turns, with each turn overlapping the preceding turn by about ¾ of its width. Bandage until the foot (not toes), ankle, and lower part of the leg are covered. Keep the toes exposed to check for circulation problems.

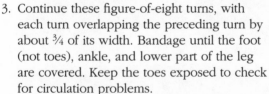

4. Secure the bandage with tape, clips, or safety pins, or tie off as described in the section on the circular bandage.

Fingertip Bandages

The fingertip bandage is particularly useful when the fingertip itself is injured. To apply a fingertip bandage:

1. Anchor the bandage at the base of the finger with a few circular turns, being careful not to wrap the bandage too tightly.

2. With your index finger of one hand, hold the bandage down at the base where it is anchored. Bring the roll of bandage up the front of the finger you are bandaging, over the fingertip, and down the back side to the base of the finger.

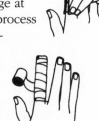

3. With your thumb, hold down the bandage at the base and repeat the back-and-forth process of bandaging over the fingertip until several layers cover the finger.

4. Starting at the base of the finger, make circular turns up the finger and back to the base to hold the bandage in place.

5. To secure the bandage, apply a piece of tape approximately 6 inches long up the side of the finger, across the tip, and down the other side of the finger. Or tie off as described in the section on the circular bandage.

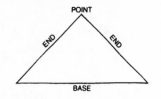

Triangular Bandages

The triangular bandage has many uses in an emergency. It can serve as a covering for a large area such as the scalp or as a sling for a broken bone, or it can be folded into a rectangular scarf and used as a circular or figure-of-eight bandage. A triangular bandage is usually made of muslin, but other material can be used. It can be easily made at home. To make a triangular bandage, cut a piece of cloth 36 to 40 inches square. Next, cut the fabric diagonally from corner to corner. Now you have two triangular bandages.

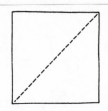

TRIANGULAR BANDAGE

A triangular bandage can be used as a sling, as a head bandage, or as a (rectangular) figure-of-eight bandage. (See illustrations on the following pages.)

Slings

To make a sling:

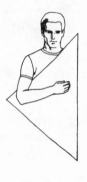

1. Place one end of the bandage over the un-injured shoulder so that the base and other end of the triangle hang down over the chest. Place the point under the elbow of the injured arm.

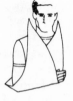

2. Elevate the hand about 4 inches above the level of the elbow and lift the lower end of the bandage up over the other shoulder.

3. Tie the two ends together at the side of the neck.

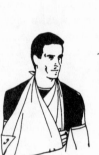

4. Fold the point forward to the front of the sling and pin it to the outside of the sling. Leave the fingers exposed.

Head Bandages

To make a head bandage:

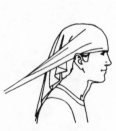

1. Place the center of the base of the triangle across the forehead so that it lies just above the eyes, with the point of the bandage down the back of the head. Bring both ends above the ears and around to the back of the head.

2. Just below the lump at the back of the head, cross the two ends over each other snugly and continue to bring the ends back around to the center of the forehead.

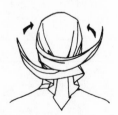

3. Tie the ends in a knot.

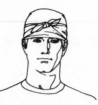

4. Tuck the point hanging down the back of the head into the fold where the bandage crosses in the back.

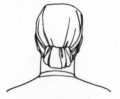

SPLINTS

Splints are used to keep an injured body part from moving, thereby easing the pain and preventing further injury. Objects that can be used for splinting include boards, straight sticks, brooms, pieces of corrugated cardboard bent to form a three-sided box, rolled newspapers or magazines, pillows, rolled blankets, oars, umbrellas, or tongue depressors (for finger injuries). The splint should extend above and below the injured area to immobilize it.

Padding such as cloth, towels, or blankets should be placed between the splint and the skin of the injured part. Splints can be tied in place with neckties, strips of cloth torn from shirts, handkerchiefs, belts, string, rope, or other suitable material. *Do not* tie the splint so tightly that the ties interfere with circulation. Swelling or bluish discoloration in the fingers or toes may indicate that the ties are too tight and need to be loosened. Also loosen splint ties if the victim experiences numbness or tingling, or if he or she cannot move the fingers or toes. Check the wrist or ankle for a pulse and loosen the ties if you can't feel a pulse.

To splint specific broken bones, see Broken Bones, p. 107.

EMERGENCY
PROCEDURES TO KNOW

Knowing how to do cardiopulmonary resuscitation (CPR) and the Heimlich maneuver can help you save a life. CPR and first-aid courses may be offered in your community by the American Red Cross or the American Heart Association, a hospital, fire department, community center, school, or employer. Ask your doctor about classes in your area and sign up today. Once you learn the CPR techniques, practice them often so you will remember how to perform them in an emergency. The CPR techniques presented here are meant to reinforce what you learn in a CPR class; they are not a substitute for the course.

CARDIOPULMONARY RESUSCITATION (CPR)*

CPR is a basic life-support technique used for a person who is not breathing and whose heart may have stopped beating. The technique allows you to perform manually the involuntary actions of the heart and lungs that provide vital blood and oxygen to all parts of the body. CPR involves opening and clearing the victim's airway (by tilting the head backward and lifting the chin), restoring breathing (by mouth-to-mouth, mouth-to-nose, or mouth-to-mouth-and-nose resuscitation), and restoring blood circulation (by external chest compressions).

---

*NOTE: There is concern among those who provide first aid—even on a one-time basis—that HIV (the virus that causes AIDS) may be contracted from a victim's body fluids. It is extremely unlikely that you will contract HIV from the blood or saliva of a person who requires mouth-to-mouth resuscitation or CPR. HIV can be passed to others through an infected person's blood and semen. The virus may be present in saliva, but cases in which it has been transmitted through saliva are unknown at present. People who regularly come in contact with blood or saliva—doctors, paramedics, other emergency department personnel, and dentists—wear protective clothing including face masks and gloves. Even among these health-care professionals, the risk of contracting HIV is extremely low.

The ABCs of CPR

A simple method of remembering the order of action to take in an emergency if the victim is not breathing or if his or her heart is not beating is the use of the term "ABCs." These letters stand for airway, breathing, and circulation, which represent the three basic steps in CPR: open and clear the victim's airway, restore breathing, and restore blood circulation.

A. Airway

The victim's airway must be clear and open in order to restore breathing. Clear the airway by doing the following:

1. Lay the victim on his or her back on a firm, flat surface such as the floor or the ground. For an infant, the hard surface may be your forearm and the palm of your hand.
2. Quickly clear the mouth and airway of any visible foreign material with your fingers and remove any loose dentures.

If there does not appear to be any neck injury:*

3. Tilt the head backward to open the airway. Do this by placing your palm on the victim's forehead and the fingers of your other hand under the bony part of the victim's chin, lifting the chin. Doing this will elevate the tongue from the back of the throat.

If you suspect an injury to the head or neck:

3. Open the airway with a procedure called the jaw thrust (see illustration on p. 32). Position yourself facing the top of the person's head, place two or three fingers of each hand under each side of his or her lower jaw, and lift the jaw upward and toward you. Try to keep the person's spine immobile and don't let the head tilt back. If the person's mouth is closed, use your thumb to pull the lower lip downward. You can use this procedure on children over 1 year.

---

*If you suspect a head, neck, or back injury—especially if the victim has fallen from a height, has fallen from a motorcycle, has been hit by a car, or has been involved in a diving accident—*and* if the victim is unconscious, *do not* move him or her. Exceptions to this rule apply only if you and the victim are in imminent danger of death, such as in or near a fire, at an accident scene in which an explosion might occur, or near a collapsing building. (See Head, Neck, and Back Injuries, p. 194.)

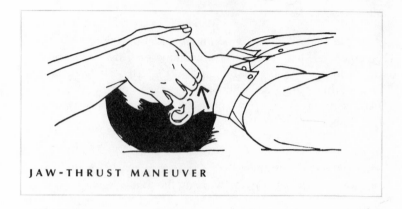

JAW-THRUST MANEUVER

For an infant under 1 year:

3. Tilt the child's head back only slightly, or the airway could be closed off. To tilt the head back, place your index finger of one hand under the child's chin and the other hand at the top of the child's head and lift the chin up toward the top of the child's head. Do not close the child's mouth or press under his or her chin or you could close off the airway.

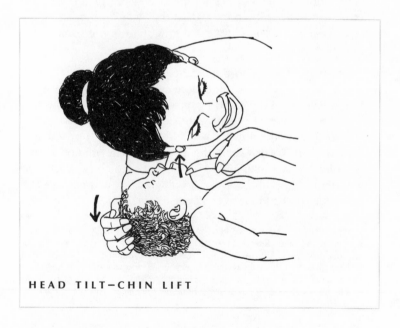

HEAD TILT—CHIN LIFT

B. Breathing

To restore breathing:

1. Be sure that the victim's head is tilted backward.
2. With the hand that is placed on the victim's forehead, pinch the victim's nostrils closed, using your thumb and index finger.
3. Open your mouth wide and take a deep breath.

If the victim is an adult or a child over 1 year:

4. Place your open mouth tightly around the victim's mouth and give two full breaths—so that air enters his or her lungs—1½ to 2 seconds per breath if the victim is an adult or a child over 8 years or 1 to 1½ seconds per breath for a child between 1 and 8 years. Remove your mouth after each breath and inhale deeply before giving the next breath.

For an infant under 1 year:

4. Place your mouth tightly over the victim's mouth and nose and blow gently at a rate of one breath every 3 seconds.

If the victim's mouth cannot be used due to an injury:

4. Lift the lower jaw to close the mouth. Open your mouth wide and take a deep breath. Place your mouth tightly around the victim's nose and blow into it. After your breath, remove your hand from the victim's mouth to allow air to escape.

5. You will feel moderate resistance when you blow. If you encounter *marked* resistance and the chest does not rise, the airway is not clear and more airway opening is needed. Place your hands under the victim's lower jaw and thrust the lower jaw up so that it juts out farther. For a child who does not have a head or neck injury, you may need to tilt the head back a little farther.

6. As you blow air into the victim's mouth, nose, or mouth and nose, watch closely to see when his or her chest rises, and stop blowing when you notice the chest is expanding.

7. Remove your mouth from the victim's mouth, nose, or mouth and nose and turn your head toward the victim's chest so that your ear is over his or her mouth. Listen for air leaving the victim's lungs and watch the chest fall. You may also feel air being exhaled from the victim's nose and mouth.

8. Continue blowing into the victim's mouth, nose, or mouth and nose at approximately 12 full breaths per minute (one breath

every 5 seconds) for a child over 8 years or an adult and 20 full breaths per minute (one breath every 3 seconds) for an infant or child up to 8 years. Provide plenty of air with each breath so that the victim's chest rises.

9. Continue breathing for the victim until he or she begins breathing on his or her own or until medical assistance arrives.

MOUTH-TO-MOUTH RESUSCITATION

Here is a summary of the steps to perform to restore breathing in a person who has stopped breathing:

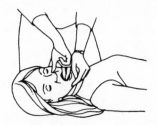

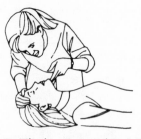

1. Make sure the victim is on a hard, flat surface. Quickly clear the mouth and airway of foreign material.

2. Tilt the victim's head backward by placing the palm of your hand on his or her forehead and the fingers of your other hand under the bony part of the chin.

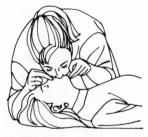

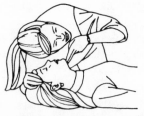

3. Pinch the victim's nostrils with your thumb and index finger. Take a deep breath. Place your mouth tightly over the victim's mouth (mouth and nose for an infant under 1 year). Give two full breaths.

4. Stop blowing when you notice the victim's chest expanding. Remove your mouth from the victim's mouth and turn your head toward the victim's chest, so that your ear is over his or her mouth. *Listen* for air being exhaled. *Watch* for the victim's chest to rise and fall. Repeat the breathing procedure.

C. Circulation

The procedure to restore blood circulation must be done in conjunction with artificial breathing. In emergency situations, restoring circulation for the victim is essential for survival, and chest compressions, as outlined on the following pages, should be attempted. If you are performing CPR, have someone else call paramedics or an ambulance. The following information includes steps for clearing the airway and restoring breathing that have been discussed previously.

CPR on an Adult

1. Assess the situation. Is the victim conscious? Gently shake him or her and ask, "Are you okay?" Do not shake or move the victim if you suspect a head or neck injury.
2. If there is no response, call to someone to get help.
3. *Look, listen,* and *feel* for breathing. Look for the victim's chest to rise and fall.
4. Open the victim's mouth and check for any foreign matter. If you see an object, remove it by sweeping your fingers across the back of the throat.

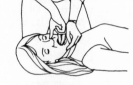

If the victim is not breathing:

5. Tilt the head backward to open the airway. Do this by placing your palm on the victim's forehead and the fingers of your other hand under the bony part of his or her chin.

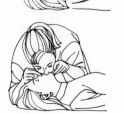

6. Pinch the victim's nose closed and blow two full breaths into his or her mouth so that the chest rises. Remove your mouth after each breath and inhale deeply before giving the next breath.

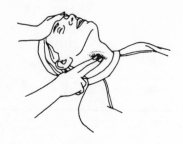

7. Check for a pulse. With the palm of one hand on the victim's forehead (to ensure that the head is tilted backward and that the airway is open), with the other hand check for a pulse on the victim's neck (carotid artery). To find the pulse in the carotid artery, move two fingers along the victim's throat to the Adam's apple. Then move these fingers off to the side of the victim's throat between the trachea (windpipe) and the muscles at the side of the neck. Press down gradually and firmly for a few seconds until you feel a pulse. *A pulse means that the heart is beating.*

If there is a pulse, but no breathing:

8. Perform mouth-to-mouth resuscitation at 12 full breaths per minute—one breath every 5 seconds until the victim starts breathing. (See p. 34.)

If there is no pulse:

8. Begin chest compressions as well. Proper hand position for chest compressions is important so that you do not damage ribs or internal organs.

To establish proper hand position for chest compressions:

1. If possible, make sure that the victim is lying on a hard, flat surface. The head should be at the same level as the rest of the body or slightly lower so that blood flow to the brain is not further reduced. If possible, slightly elevate the legs, which will help blood flow back to the heart. *Move quickly so that valuable time is not lost.*

2. Kneel near the victim's chest and, with two fingers, locate his or her rib cage on the side closest to you. Move your fingers up the center of the victim's chest to the notch where the ribs meet the breastbone (sternum). With your fingers on this notch, place the heel of your other hand two finger-widths above your fingers.

3. Remove your fingers from the notch of the breastbone and place them on top of your other hand. The fingers of both hands should be interlaced. Do not allow your fingers to rest on the ribs—press down with the heel of your hand only.

4. While kneeling, position your shoulders directly over the victim so that all of your weight is forced down, through the heel of your hand, onto the victim's chest. Straighten your arms and lock your elbows. Use your arms to exert pressure.

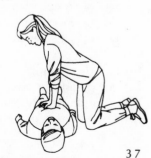

37

To perform compressions:

5. Push down on the chest 15 times. With each compression, push down quickly and forcefully to a depth of 1½ to 2 inches. Let the chest rise after each compression, *but do not remove your hands from the chest.* The compression movements should be smooth, not jerky. Perform the compressions rhythmically by counting out loud: "1 and, 2 and, 3 and, 4 and, 5 and, 6 and, 7 and, 8 and, 9 and, 10 and, 11 and, 12 and, 13 and, 14 and, 15 and."

6. Release your hands from the victim's chest and open the airway by tilting the head and chin backward.

7. Pinch the victim's nostrils shut with your thumb and index finger. Blow two slow, full breaths into the victim's mouth so that the chest rises.

8. Reposition your hands on the victim's chest and repeat the cycle of 15 compressions and two breaths until you have performed four complete cycles.

9. Determine if the victim's pulse has returned. To do this, feel the victim's carotid artery in the neck. *Do not, however, interrupt CPR for longer than 7 seconds.* To find the pulse in the carotid artery, move two fingers along the victim's throat to the Adam's apple. Then move these fingers off to the side of the victim's throat between the trachea (windpipe) and the muscles at the side of the neck. Press down gradually and firmly until you feel a pulse. *A pulse means that the heart is beating.*

If there is a pulse but no breathing:

10. Perform mouth-to-mouth resuscitation at 12 breaths per minute—one breath every 5 seconds until the person starts breathing. (See p. 34.)

If there is no pulse:

10. Repeat the cycles of 15 compressions and two breaths. The rate of compressions should be about 80 to 100 per minute. Continue CPR until the victim begins breathing and his or her heart begins beating or until professional help arrives.

N O T E : *If vomiting occurs during CPR,* turn the victim on his or her side (rolling the whole body as a unit) and clear out the mouth with your fingers. Return the victim to his or her back and tilt the head backward to open the airway. Resume CPR if necessary.

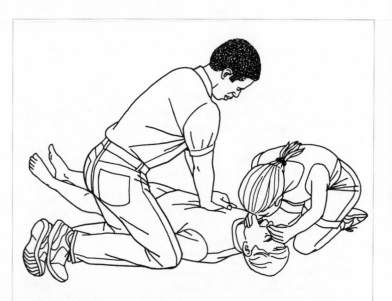

CPR WITH TWO RESCUERS

CPR can be done by two rescuers who can share the tasks. One rescuer kneels at the victim's side performing chest compressions at a rate of 80 to 100 per minute. This rescuer pauses after every fifth compression to allow the second rescuer, who is kneeling at the victim's head, to perform one slow, full breath. The second rescuer checks frequently for a pulse to ensure that the compressions are adequate to pump blood. The CPR rhythm is five compressions for every breath.

CPR on a Child 1 to 8 Years:

(For large children or for those over 8 years, use the steps outlined for an adult.)

1. Assess the situation. Is the victim conscious? Gently shake him or her and ask, "Are you okay?" Do not shake or move the child if you suspect a head or neck injury.
2. If there is no response, call to someone to get help.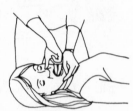
3. *Look, listen,* and *feel* for breathing. Look for the child's chest to rise and fall.
4. Open the child's mouth and check for any foreign matter. If you see an object, remove it by sweeping your fingers across the back of the throat.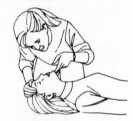

If the child is not breathing:
5. Tilt the head backward to open the airway. Do this by placing your palm on the child's forehead and the fingers of your other hand under the bony part of his or her chin. You can also use the jaw-thrust procedure described on p. 32.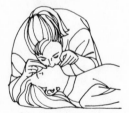
6. With the hand that is on the child's forehead, pinch the child's nostrils closed with your thumb and index finger. Place your mouth over the child's mouth and blow two full breaths so that his or her chest rises. Remove your mouth after each breath and inhale deeply before giving the next breath.
7. Check for a pulse. With the palm of one hand on the child's forehead (to ensure that the head is tilted backward and that the airway is open), with the other hand check for a pulse on his or her neck (carotid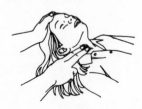

artery). To find the pulse in the carotid artery, move two fingers along the victim's throat to the Adam's apple. Then move these fingers off to the side of the child's throat, between the trachea (windpipe) and the muscles at the side of the neck. Press down gradually and gently for a few seconds until you feel a pulse. *A pulse means that the heart is beating.*

If there is a pulse but no breathing:

8. Perform mouth-to-mouth resuscitation at 20 breaths per minute (one breath every 3 seconds) until the child starts breathing. (See p. 34.)

If there is no pulse:

8. Begin chest compressions as well. Proper hand position for chest compressions is important so that you do not damage ribs or internal organs.

To establish proper hand position for chest compressions:

1. If possible, make sure that the victim is lying on a hard, flat surface. The head should be at the same level as the rest of the body or slightly lower so that blood flow to the brain is not further reduced. If possible, slightly elevate the legs, which will help blood flow back to the head. *Move quickly so that valuable time is not lost.*

2. Kneel near the victim's chest and, with two fingers, locate his or her rib cage on the side closest to you. Move your fingers up the center of the victim's chest to the notch where the ribs meet the breastbone (sternum). With your fingers on this notch, place the heel of your other hand two finger-widths above your fingers. 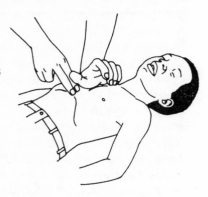 Remove your fingers from the notch. Use one hand only for compressions, pressing down with just the heel of the hand and keeping your fingers from resting on the child's ribs (as shown).

41

3. While kneeling, position your shoulders directly over the victim so that all of your weight is forced down, through the heel of your hand only, onto the victim's chest. Straighten your arm and lock your elbow. Use your arm to exert pressure.

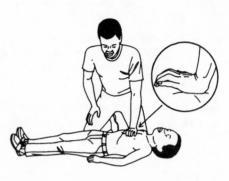

To perform compressions:

4. Push down on the chest five times. With each compression push down quickly and forcefully to a depth of 1 to 1½ inches. Let the chest rise after each compression, *but do not remove your hand from the chest.* The compression movements should be smooth, not jerky. Perform them rhythmically by counting out loud: "1 and, 2 and, 3 and, 4 and, 5 and."

5. Release your hand from the child's chest and open the airway by tilting the head and chin backward.

6. Blow two slow, full breaths into the child's mouth and nose so that the chest rises.

7. Reposition your hand on the child's chest and repeat the cycle of five compressions and one breath until you have performed 20 complete cycles of five compressions and one breath. Each breath should last about 1 second and the rate of compressions should be 100 per minute.

8. Determine if the child's pulse has returned. To do this, feel the child's carotid artery in the neck. *Do not, however, interrupt CPR for longer than 7 seconds.* To find the pulse in the carotid artery, move two fingers along the child's throat to the Adam's apple. Then move these fingers off to the side of the child's throat between the trachea (windpipe) and the muscles at the side of the neck. Press down gradually and gently until you feel a pulse. *A pulse means that the heart is beating.*

If there is a pulse, but no breathing:

9. Perform mouth-to-mouth-and-nose resuscitation at 20 breaths per minute (one breath every 3 seconds) until the child starts breathing.

If there is no pulse:

9. Repeat the five compressions and one breath. Continue CPR until the victim begins breathing and his or her heart begins beating or until professional help arrives.

N O T E : *If vomiting occurs during CPR,* turn the victim on his or her side (rolling the victim's whole body as a unit) and clear out the mouth with your fingers. Return the victim to his or her back and tilt the head backward to open the airway. Resume mouth-to-mouth resuscitation and CPR if necessary.

CPR on an Infant Under 1 Year:

1. Assess the situation. Is the infant conscious? Gently shake him or her and shout to elicit a cry or other response. Do not shake or move the child if you suspect a head or neck injury.
2. If there is no response, call to someone to get help.
3. *Look, listen,* and *feel* for breath-
ing. Look for the infant's chest
to rise and fall.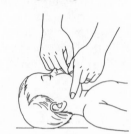
4. Open the infant's mouth and
check for any foreign matter in
the mouth. If you see an object, remove it by sweeping
your fingers across the back of
the throat.

If the infant is not breathing:

5. Tilt the head backward slightly to open the airway. Do this by placing your palm on the infant's forehead and the fingers of your other hand under the bony part of the infant's chin. *Do not extend the head too far back. Doing so may close off the airway.*

6. Place your mouth over the infant's mouth and nose and
blow two breaths so that his
or her chest rises. Do not
blow air as forcefully as for an
adult. Remove your mouth
after each breath and inhale
deeply before giving the next
breath.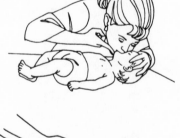

7. Check for a pulse. With
the palm of one hand on
the infant's forehead (to
ensure that the head is
tilted backward and that
the airway is open), place
the index and middle
fingers of your other hand
on the infant's brachial
artery on the inside of the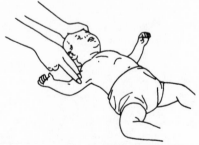
upper arm and rest your thumb against the outside of the
arm. *A pulse means that the heart is beating.*

If there is a pulse but no breathing:

8. Perform mouth-to-mouth-and-nose resuscitation at 20 breaths per minute (one breath every 3 seconds) until the infant starts breathing.

If there is no pulse:

8. Begin chest compressions as well. Proper finger position is important so that you do not damage ribs or internal organs. (See below.)

To establish proper finger position on the chest for CPR:

1. If possible, place the infant on his or her back on a hard, flat surface. The head should be at the same level as the rest of the body or slightly lower so that blood flow to the brain is not further reduced. *Move quickly so that valuable time is not lost.*
2. Place the palm of your hand on the infant's forehead and tilt the head back. *Do not extend the head too far back. Doing so may close off the airway.* With your other hand, locate an imaginary line between the infant's nipples on the breastbone. Place two fingers one finger-width below this line on the breastbone. Try to keep your palm in position on the infant's forehead and your fingers in position on the infant's chest throughout compressions. You may find it easier to steady the infant's head and body during compressions by placing your fingers and thumb on either side of the infant's head (as shown).

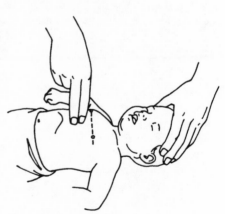

To perform compressions:

3. Using two fingers, push down on the infant's chest five times. With each compression, push down to a depth of ½ to 1 inch. Let the chest rise after each compression, *but do not remove your fingers from the chest.* The compression movements

should be smooth, not jerky. Perform them rhythmically by counting out loud: "1 and, 2 and, 3 and, 4 and, 5 and."

4. After five compressions, blow air once into the infant's mouth and nose. Perform 10 complete cycles of five compressions and one breath.

5. Determine if the infant's pulse has returned. To do this, feel for a pulse in the brachial artery, located on the inside of the upper arm between the elbow and shoulder (see p. 18). *A pulse means that the heart is beating. Do not, however, interrupt CPR for longer than 7 seconds.*

If there is a pulse but no breathing:

6. Perform mouth-to-mouth-and-nose resuscitation at 20 breaths per minute (one breath every 3 seconds) until the infant starts breathing.

If there is no pulse:

6. Repeat the five compressions and one breath. The rate of compressions should be at least 100 per minute. Continue CPR until the infant begins breathing and his or her heart begins beating or until professional help arrives.

N O T E : *If vomiting occurs during CPR,* turn the infant on his or her side, and clear out the mouth with your fingers. Return the infant to his or her back and tilt the head backward to open the airway. Resume mouth-to-mouth-and-nose resuscitation and CPR if necessary.

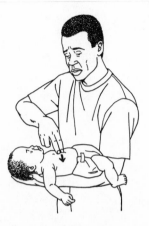

ALTERNATIVE POSITION FOR CPR ON INFANT

An alternative position for giving CPR to a small infant, if you cannot find a flat surface to lay the infant on, or if you need to be moving, is to hold the child on your forearm, supporting his or her head with the palm of your hand and keeping the head level with the torso. Perform chest compressions with your other hand, following the CPR instructions in steps 1 through 8 on pp. 44–45.

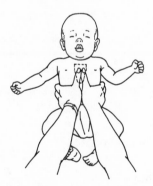

ALTERNATIVE TECHNIQUE FOR DOING CHEST COMPRESSIONS ON INFANT

A newer technique for doing chest compressions on an infant (3 months old or younger) who is lying on a firm surface is to encircle the child's chest with both hands and place both of your thumbs on the middle of the infant's breastbone at the nipple line. For each compression, press your thumbs down into the breastbone ½ to 1 inch, following the CPR instructions in steps 1 through 6 on pp. 45–46.

CPR DOS AND DON'TS

The success of your CPR efforts will depend in large part on performing the CPR technique properly. Below is a list of reminders to help you. Remember: Perform chest compressions only if you do not feel a pulse.

DO

- Kneel alongside the victim to perform chest compressions. Straighten your arms, lock your elbows, and use your arms to exert pressure.
- Perform quick, forceful compressions straight down on the chest.
- Interlock fingers and use the heel of the bottom hand only for compressions. For children between 1 and 8 years, use only one hand. For infants under 1 year, use only the index and middle fingers of one hand.
- Keep your hands (or fingers) in place on the chest while performing compressions.

DON'T

- Don't rock back and forth or sit on your heels while performing compressions. (Blood will not be pumped out of the heart effectively.)
- Don't roll your hands on the victim's chest.
- Don't lift your hands off the victim's chest or "bounce" your hands on the chest while performing compressions.
- Don't allow your fingers to rest or exert pressure on the victim's rib cage.

CPR REMINDERS

	Adults	Children 1 to 8 Years	Infants Under 1 Year
Check for pulse on:	side of neck (carotid artery)	side of neck (carotid artery)	inner part of upper arm (brachial artery)
If there is a pulse but no breathing, give one breath every:	5 seconds (12 per minute)	3 seconds (20 per minute)	3 seconds (20 per minute)
If there is no pulse, begin CPR by:	tracing the victim's ribs to the notch at the center of the chest and placing the heel of your other hand two finger-widths above the notch	tracing the victim's ribs to the notch at the center of the chest and placing the heel of your other hand two finger-widths above the notch	placing two fingers one finger-width below an imaginary line between the nipples
Push down on (compress) the chest with:	the heel of one hand on the breastbone, with the other hand on top of it, fingers interlaced	the heel of one hand only on the child's breastbone	two or three fingers on the breastbone
Compress the chest to a depth of:	1½–2 inches	1–1½ inches	½–1 inch
Number of compressions to breaths:	15:2	5:1	5:1

GLOSSARY OF CPR TERMS

ABCs A term that describes the three basic steps in CPR: maintain an open airway, restore breathing, and restore circulation, if necessary.

Brachial artery One of the main arteries in the body, found on the inside of the upper arm, between the elbow and shoulder. A rescuer can feel for a pulse—primarily in infants under 1 year —by gently pressing on this artery.

Cardiac arrest A critical medical condition in which the heart has stopped beating.

Carotid artery One of the main arteries in the body, found on either side of the neck. A rescuer can feel for a pulse—primarily in children over 1 year and adults—by gently, but firmly, pressing on this artery.

Compressions Downward thrusts on the chest with the hands. Compressing or pushing down on the chest, like pressing water out of a sponge, pushes blood out of the heart to all parts of the body. Releasing pressure on the chest allows the rib cage to expand and, again similar to the dynamics of a sponge, draws blood into the heart.

CPR Cardiopulmonary resuscitation, which means, literally, heart and lung revival. The process of clearing the airway, restoring breathing, and restoring blood circulation.

Pulse The "wave" of blood flowing through arteries and veins that is in rhythm with the beating of the heart. When a rescuer feels for a pulse in one of the main arteries in the body, he or she is determining if the heart is beating.

Respiration The process of breathing.

Resuscitation The attempt to restore breathing and, if necessary, blood circulation in a victim. This is done by mouth-to-mouth, mouth-to-nose, or mouth-to-mouth-and-nose respirations and by chest compressions.

Ventilations The process of breathing air into a victim's lungs. This is done in mouth-to-mouth, mouth-to-nose, or mouth-to-mouth-and-nose resuscitation.

HEIMLICH MANEUVER FOR CHOKING

The Heimlich maneuver (abdominal thrust) is the recommended method to use when a person is choking. Back blows—hitting the victim forcefully and repeatedly between the shoulder blades with the palm of your hand—are used on adults and children only if the Heimlich maneuver has not been effective in dislodging a foreign object from the windpipe (trachea).

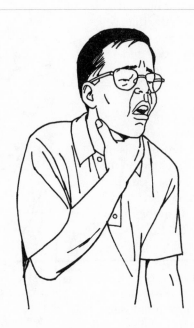

UNIVERSAL CHOKING SIGN
A person who is choking will involuntarily grasp his or her neck.

Heimlich Maneuver on an Adult or a Child Over 1 Year:

If the victim can speak, cough, or breathe:
This means that he or she is moving air through the airway. Do not interfere in any way with his or her efforts to cough out a swallowed or partially swallowed object.

If the victim cannot breathe:

1. Stand behind him or her and place your fist with the thumb side against his or her stomach slightly above the navel and below the ribs and breastbone. Be careful not to touch the breastbone.

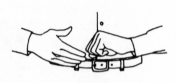

2. Hold your fist with your other hand and give several quick, forceful upward thrusts. This maneuver increases pressure in the abdomen, which pushes up the diaphragm. This, in turn, increases the air pressure in the lungs and will often force out the object from the windpipe. Do not squeeze on the person's ribs with your arms—use only your fist in the abdomen. It may be necessary to repeat the Heimlich maneuver 6 to 10 times.

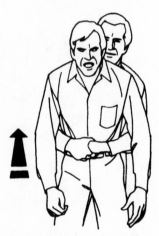

If the victim is lying down:
Turn the victim on his or her back. Straddle the victim and put the heel of your hand on his or her stomach, slightly above the navel and below the ribs. Put your free hand on top of your other hand to provide additional force. Keep your elbows straight. Give several quick, forceful downward and forward thrusts toward the person's head in an attempt to dislodge the object. Doing so will increase pressure in the abdomen, forcing pressure into the lungs to expel the object out of the windpipe and into the mouth. It may be necessary to repeat the procedure 6 to 10 times.

If you get no results:

Repeat the Heimlich maneuver until the victim coughs up the object or becomes unconscious. Look to see if the object appears in the victim's mouth or at the top of the throat. Use your fingers to pull the object out.

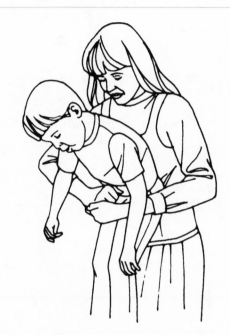

HEIMLICH MANEUVER ON A CHILD OVER 1 YEAR

Stand behind the child with your arms around his or her waist. Place the thumb side of your fist against the child's stomach slightly above the navel and below the ribs and breastbone. Be careful not to touch the breastbone. Hold your fist with your other hand and give several quick, forceful upward thrusts. It may be necessary to repeat the procedure 6 to 10 times.

Heimlich Maneuver on an Infant Under 1 Year:

1. Place the infant face down across your forearm with his or her head slightly lower than the trunk. Support the head by firmly holding the infant's jaw. Rest your forearm on your thigh and give five forceful back blows with the heel of your hand between the infant's shoulder blades pressing

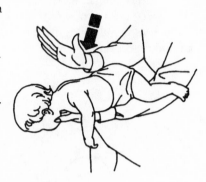

downward and toward the child's head. The blows should be more gentle than those for an adult.

2. If unsuccessful, turn the infant over onto his or her back, keeping the head lower than the trunk. Give five quick thrusts on the chest. To do this, place two fingers one finger-width below an imaginary line joining the nipples. Push downward. Thrusts should be more gentle than those for an adult.

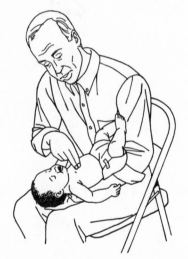

3. If necessary, repeat both procedures.

Special Circumstances

If the Choking Victim Is Unconscious or Becomes Unconscious

1. Place the victim on his or her back on a rigid surface, such as the ground.

2. Open the victim's airway by extending the head backward. To do this, place the palm of your hand on the victim's forehead and the fingers of your other hand under the bony part of the chin. Attempt to restore breathing with mouth-to-mouth resuscitation. (See p. 34.)

3. If still unsuccessful, and with the victim on his or her back, begin the Heimlich maneuver by putting the heel of one hand on the victim's stomach slightly above the navel and below the ribs. Put your free hand on top of your other hand to provide additional force. 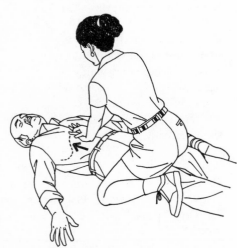 Keep your elbows straight. Give several quick, forceful, downward and forward thrusts toward the head.

4. If these procedures fail, grasp the victim's lower jaw and tongue with one hand and lift up to remove the tongue from the back of the throat. Place the index finger of the other hand inside the victim's mouth alongside the cheek. Slide your fingers down into the throat to the base of the victim's tongue.

   Carefully sweep your fingers along the back of the throat to dislodge the object. Bring your fingers out along the inside of the other cheek. Be careful not to push the object farther down the victim's throat. If a foreign body comes within reach, grasp and remove it. *Do not* attempt to remove the foreign object with any type of instrument or forceps unless you are trained to do so.

5. Repeat all of the above steps until the object is dislodged or medical assistance arrives. Do not give up!

If the Choking Victim Is Very Overweight or Pregnant

1. Stand behind the victim and place your fist on the middle of the breastbone in the chest, but not over the ribs. Put your other hand on top of it. Give several quick, forceful movements. *Do not* squeeze with your arms—use just your fist.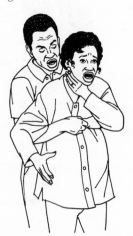

2. If this procedure does not work, stand behind the victim and support his or her chest with one hand. With the heel of the other hand give several quick blows on the back between the victim's shoulder blades.

If You Are Alone and Choking

1. Place your fist on your stomach slightly above your navel and below your breastbone. Place your other hand on top of your fist. Give yourself several quick, forceful upward abdominal thrusts.

2. If this procedure does not work, press your stomach forcefully over a chair, table, or railing.

PART II

ALPHABETICAL LISTING OF INJURIES AND ILLNESSES

There are hundreds of causes of abdominal pain, some of which can indicate serious medical problems that require immediate medical care. Abdominal pain in children is common and is usually not serious unless it lasts longer than an hour or is accompanied by other symptoms. But severe abdominal pain in infants and young children can indicate a serious medical disorder that requires immediate medical attention. For both adults and children, if symptoms are severe or persist, seek medical attention promptly. A person with severe abdominal pain should never be given an enema, a laxative, medication, food, or liquids (including water) without a doctor's advice, since doing so may aggravate the problem or cause a complication.

ABDOMINAL PAIN IN ADULTS

An adult who has abdominal pain under any of the following conditions requires immediate medical attention and should be taken to a hospital emergency department:

- Recent abdominal surgery or endoscopy (a procedure to diagnose or treat digestive disorders through a viewing tube called an endoscope)
- Pain that is focused in one specific area of the abdomen
- Pain that begins intermittently in a general area around the navel and later moves to the lower right part of the abdomen
- Pain that travels to the back or shoulder area
- Pain that is accompanied by fever, sweating, blood in stool, black stool, or blood in urine
- Pain that becomes suddenly severe and intolerable or that wakes a person from sleep
- Severe pain in the side or back that radiates to the groin
- Pain during pregnancy or with abnormal vaginal bleeding
- Pain that is accompanied by dry mouth, sunken eyes, dizzy

feeling when standing, or decreased urination (symptoms of dehydration)
- Pain that is accompanied by difficulty breathing
- Pain that is associated with an injury to the abdomen
- Pain that is accompanied by vomiting blood or a greenish-brown fluid

ABDOMINAL PAIN IN INFANTS AND YOUNG CHILDREN UP TO ABOUT AGE 5

An infant with abdominal pain will usually cry loudly, bending the legs and drawing the knees toward his or her chest. A young child should be taken to a hospital emergency department if he or she has abdominal pain under any of the following conditions:

- Forceful vomiting right after feedings in a very young infant (usually between 3 and 6 weeks old)
- Pain that occurs suddenly, subsides, and then recurs without warning
- Pain that is accompanied by red or purple, jellylike stool; blood in stool; or mucus in stool
- Pain that is accompanied by greenish-brown vomit
- Swollen abdomen that feels hard to the touch
- A hard lump in the scrotum, groin, or lower abdomen

See Also: Diarrhea, p. 148; Food Poisoning, p. 185; Miscarriage, p. 219; Pregnancy Danger Signs, p. 228; Vomiting, p. 262; Wounds (Abdominal Wounds), p. 264.

Reported cases of child abuse, and abuse of other individuals, such as spouses and the elderly, have risen dramatically. Abuse can take many forms—emotional, physical, or sexual—or can involve neglect. In most instances, the abuser is a parent or other family member, a neighbor, or some other adult. People who abuse were often abused themselves as children.

Making an assessment that abuse has occurred or is occurring can be difficult. Always call the police if you suspect with good reason that a child or other person is being abused or is in danger of losing his or her life. If you are abusing a child or other person, help is available to you. Call a child abuse hotline or other community agency that offers counseling.

SYMPTOMS

Some symptoms and signs of abuse are more obvious than others. If a person has been physically abused, he or she may exhibit any or all of the following:

- Frequent complaints of pain
- Frequent broken bones
- Unexplained cuts, bruises, or burn marks
- Bleeding
- Multiple injuries on different parts of the body that are healing in different stages
- Withdrawal, depression, or inattentiveness
- Excessive aggression

If a child has been sexually abused, he or she may exhibit any or all of the following:

- Complaints of pain when urinating
- Unusual fear of adults

INJURIES AND ILLNESSES

61

- Injury to genital or rectal area
- Difficulty walking or sitting
- Withdrawal, depression, or inattentiveness
- Excessive masturbation
- Promiscuous or sexually precocious behavior

If a person (usually a child or elderly person) has been neglected, he or she may exhibit any or all of the following:

- An unkempt appearance; poor hygiene
- Lack of appropriate medical care for a chronic illness or injury; lack of required immunizations
- Malnourishment
- Lack of appropriate supervision

WHAT TO DO

For a victim of physical or sexual abuse:
1. Treat noticeable injuries, such as cuts, bruises, or burns.
2. Do not allow the victim to take a shower, bathe, brush his or her teeth, or eat or drink anything until he or she has been examined professionally; this preserves any evidence of abuse.
3. Comfort the victim as much as possible.
4. Believe the victim.
5. Do not leave the victim alone.
6. Call 911 (or your local emergency number) or take the victim to a hospital emergency department or doctor's office immediately.

For a victim of negligence:
1. Do not directly confront the person you suspect of negligence.
2. Contact a local service agency such as a child protective services agency, a senior agency or aging department, welfare department, public health authorities, or the police. Professionals in these organizations are trained to help people who are the victims of negligence and their families; they will keep your information confidential and anonymous. If your claim later turns out to be unwarranted, you cannot legally be held responsible for providing the information in good faith.

IF A RAPE HAS OCCURRED, DO NOT ALLOW THE VICTIM TO:

Change clothes.   Take a shower.   Brush his or her teeth.   Eat or drink.

BE SURE TO:

Call the police.   Call a relative or friend to assist you.   Call a doctor, a hospital emergency department, or an abuse hotline.

INJURIES AND ILLNESSES

When you seek medical treatment for a victim of sexual or physical abuse, he or she will probably be given a private room or a secluded area at the physician's office or hospital emergency department. A social worker, police officer, and medical personnel may all be present to help. You or the victim may be asked to describe several times what happened and to give a description of the abuser.

A physician will recommend that the victim have a complete physical examination. The exam is performed to protect the person from disease and to support possible criminal charges of rape or other physical abuse. The exam will include taking samples from the mouth, vagina, and rectum and testing for sexually transmitted infections (such as HIV, chlamydia, gonorrhea, or syphilis) and for a pre-existing pregnancy. The tests will determine the victim's health status at the time the incident occurred.

The victim will be advised to seek follow-up medical treatment, depending upon the injuries and test results. Medical personnel may advise the victim to seek counseling for assistance in handling the emotional aspects of physical abuse or rape. Doctors also recommend that the siblings of an abused child be examined within 24 hours.

ALTITUDE SICKNESS

Altitude sickness is caused by the lack of oxygen in the air and decreased barometric pressure at high altitudes (above 8,000 feet).

SYMPTOMS

Altitude sickness can cause any or all of the following symptoms, usually within 12 to 24 hours after a person has arrived at a high altitude:

- Headache
- Extreme tiredness
- Light-headedness; fainting
- Feeling unable to catch one's breath (sometimes causing the person to try to breathe in more air, causing hyperventilation)
- Dry cough
- Pain in the chest; tightness in the throat
- Restlessness; inability to sleep
- Nausea; vomiting
- Fast heart rate
- Hallucinations
- Panic

> **WARNING**
>
> LIFE-THREATENING SYMPTOMS
>
> If a person experiences any of the following symptoms while at a high altitude, seek medical attention immediately:
>
> - Difficulty breathing
> - Chest pain
> - Confusion
> - Decreased consciousness
> - Loss of balance

If the victim is not breathing:

1. Maintain an open airway; restore breathing and circulation if necessary. (See pp. 31–50.)
2. Seek immediate medical attention.

If the victim is breathing on his or her own:

1. Do not breathe more air, by mouth-to-mouth resuscitation, into his or her lungs.
2. Keep the victim quiet and at rest until he or she can catch his or her breath. It is *very* important for you and others to remain calm, so that the victim will remain calm, which conserves oxygen and energy. Have the victim breathe air from an auxiliary oxygen source, if available.
3. Do not continue climbing. The victim may need to return to a lower altitude of 1,800 feet or less. *Do not* send the victim off alone. Stay with him or her.
4. Suggest that the victim seek medical treatment, even after he or she has recovered and feels fine. Treatment with oxygen and medication may be necessary.

Preventing Altitude Sickness

If you have emphysema, heart disease, sickle cell anemia, epilepsy, uncontrolled high blood pressure, or have had a stroke, you may be at increased risk of altitude sickness and should talk to your doctor if you are planning to visit a high altitude. The following steps can help you avoid altitude sickness if you are traveling by air, mountain climbing, or visiting a place located at an altitude higher than you're used to:

- Take the over-the-counter decongestant pseudoephedrine half an hour before traveling by air (120 milligrams for adults). Ask your doctor if you can give it to your child before traveling and the recommended dosage for your child's size or age.
- Ask your doctor about taking acetazolamide or dexamethasone to prevent altitude sickness.
- Avoid alcohol, sedative drugs, and cigarettes for the first 2 days you are at an altitude higher than you're used to.

- Drink plenty of noncaffeinated fluids to avoid dehydration.
- Eat a diet high in carbohydrates (70 percent or more of total calories).
- Avoid strenuous exercise at high altitudes.
- If you are mountain climbing, gradually get your body acclimated to a higher altitude by climbing no more than 3,000 feet in 1 day and sleeping at the new altitude for two or three nights before continuing your ascent.
- If you are pregnant and not used to high altitudes, avoid altitudes over 13,000 feet. Check with your doctor.

INJURIES AND ILLNESSES

AMPUTATION OF SMALLER BODY PARTS

Smaller body parts—especially a fingertip, nose, ear, or penis—are easier to save and reattach when amputated than larger body parts, such as limbs. To keep an amputated part viable, it must be kept adequately cool, at a temperature of about 38°F, until a doctor can reattach it. When kept at a low temperature, muscle can survive for up to 12 hours; bone and skin can survive for up to 24 hours.

WHAT TO DO

1. Rinse the amputated body part with water or saline solution. *Do not* scrub it or use soap.
2. Wrap the amputated part in gauze or a clean cloth soaked in saline solution or water.
3. Place the part in a dry, plastic, waterproof bag.
4. Submerge the plastic bag and its contents in ice water, preferably in a polystyrene plastic container. Make sure that the ice does not come in direct contact with the amputated part.
5. Transport the injured person and the amputated part immediately to the nearest emergency department.

SEVERED LIMBS

A severed limb is a serious emergency and requires prompt medical attention. A victim who has a severed limb, such as a finger, hand, arm, or foot, may be bleeding profusely and have other problems that will need to be treated. With loss of a limb, the first medical concern is saving the person's life. The second concern is successfully reattaching the severed limb. The leg is the most difficult to reattach successfully.

WHAT TO DO

1. Call 911 (or your local emergency number). Maintain an open airway. Restore breathing and circulation if necessary. (See pp. 31–50.)
2. Treat for bleeding. (See p. 96.)
3. If the victim is vomiting, turn the victim on his or her side or turn the head sideways, *only if you do not suspect a neck injury,* so that he or she does not choke on the vomit.

To save the severed limb:

1. *After* you have cared for the victim, rinse the limb with cool water (do not use soap). Place the limb in a clean plastic bag, garbage bag, or other suitable container to keep the limb from drying out and to prevent contamination.
2. Pack ice around the limb on the *outside* of the bag or container to keep the limb cold. The ice must not touch the limb directly and the limb should not soak in ice or water. If a second bag or container is available, the ice should be placed in this bag. Then place the bag with the limb in it in the bag of ice. Keeping the limb cold decreases its need for oxygen and can keep it viable for up to 18 hours.
3. If you are transporting the victim to the hospital yourself, call the hospital to notify them of the severed limb. This will give the hospital time to prepare for the victim's arrival. If the hospital is not equipped to perform surgical reattachment, the staff often can make arrangements and will direct you to a hospital that is able to perform this procedure.

INJURIES AND ILLNESSES

ASTHMA

Asthma is a condition resulting from a gradual or sudden narrowing of the airways in the lungs, causing difficulty in breathing. Breathing may be especially difficult when exhaling. Often, but not always, an attack results from exposure to something to which the victim is allergic. However, infections (bronchitis), exercise, cold weather, inhaled irritants in the air, or emotional factors can also lead to an attack. If you have asthma, you can swim but, if you use an inhaler regularly, you should always leave it in an easy-to-reach spot by the water.

SYMPTOMS

An asthma attack can cause any or all of the following symptoms:

- Difficulty in exhaling (you might hear a wheezing or whistling sound as air is forced out through narrow airways)
- Always sitting upright (because doing so makes it easier for the victim to breathe)
- Nervousness; tenseness; fright
- Coughing
- Perspiration on forehead
- Choking sensation
- Vomiting
- Fever
- Bluish tinge to the skin in severe attacks (due to the lack of adequate oxygen intake)

WHAT TO DO

If this is the first episode of suspected (but undiagnosed) asthma:
Seek medical attention immediately. Report all details of the attack. If you can't reach a doctor, take the victim to the nearest

hospital emergency department. Comfort and reassure the victim, particularly a child who may be frightened by the experience, since emotional stress may make asthma worse. Keep the victim in a sitting position—don't force him or her to lie down.

> **WARNING**
>
> RESPIRATORY FAILURE
>
> If the victim tries to pull up the shoulders and chin to expand the chest to get air, *seek medical attention at once.* Call paramedics or go to the nearest hospital emergency department. The victim may be near respiratory failure and could collapse.

If the person has had attacks before:
Give him or her prescribed medications according to the instructions on the container. Do not give anything else without a physician's advice. Report the attack to the victim's physician.

If the symptoms continue and one or more of the following happens, seek medical attention immediately:
• Failure to improve with medication
• Difficulty inhaling or inability to exhale (breathing becomes barely audible)
• Inability to cough or talk
• Increased bluish tinge to skin, especially around the mouth or in nail beds
• Increased pulse rate to more than 120 beats per minute in an adult at rest
• Increased breathing rate of more than 30 breaths per minute in an adult at rest
• Increased anxiety; sweating
• Constant cough
• Flaring of nostrils in children
• Grunting in infants
• Inability to breathe when lying down

INJURIES AND ILLNESS

BITES AND STINGS

ANIMAL BITES

Animal bites can result in serious infections—including rabies and tetanus—as well as in tissue damage. Pit bulls, German shepherds, and mixed-breed dogs account for a large percentage of bites. Raccoons, skunks, foxes, and bats are the major carriers of rabies.

WHAT TO DO

1. Immediately clean the wound thoroughly with a 1- to 5-percent solution of povidone-iodine or with soap and running water for 5 minutes or more to wash out contaminating organisms. *Do not* put medication, antiseptics, or home remedies on the wound.
2. Put a sterile bandage or clean, dry cloth over the wound. If it is bleeding, apply pressure to the wound for 5 minutes or until the bleeding stops.
3. Seek medical attention promptly, particularly for a bite on the face, neck, or hands, which can develop into a serious infection. If some skin tissue, such as a part of an ear or a nose, is bitten off, bring it to the hospital emergency department or doctor's office with the victim. (See Amputations, p. 68.)
4. If you suspect that an animal has rabies, notify the local police, health department, or animal warden immediately. It is very important to catch and confine any animal that has bitten someone, so that it can be observed and evaluated for rabies. *Do not* attempt to catch the animal yourself.

Avoiding Animal Bites

Here are some steps you can take to avoid animal bites:

- Don't tease, provoke, or surprise an animal, especially when it is resting or eating.
- Don't have wild animals as pets.
- Don't make any sudden moves or gestures toward a strange animal.
- If confronted by an animal, back away slowly and calmly.

HUMAN BITES

Any human bite that breaks the skin needs immediate medical treatment. Human bites can lead to serious infections from bacteria or viruses that may contaminate the wound. However, bites are not considered a route of transmission of the AIDS virus. A bite on the hand can cause loss of the use of the fingers and hand.

WHAT TO DO

1. Immediately clean the wound thoroughly with a 1- to 5-percent solution of povidone-iodine or with soap and running water for 5 minutes or more to wash out contaminating organisms. *Do not* put medication, antiseptics, or home remedies on the wound.
2. Put a sterile bandage or clean, dry cloth over the wound. If it is bleeding, apply pressure to the wound for 5 minutes or until the bleeding stops.
3. Seek medical attention promptly, particularly for a bite on the face, neck, or hands, which can develop into a serious infection. If some skin tissue, such as a part of an ear or a nose, is bitten off, bring it to the hospital emergency department or doctor's office with the victim. (See Amputations, p. 68.)

INSECT STINGS

Though most insect stings cause only local reactions (redness, swelling), some can be life-threatening if the victim is allergic to the insect's venom. Insect stings cause more deaths per year than snakebites. The most common stinging insects are honeybees, hornets, wasps, yellow jackets, bumblebees, and fire ants. (See Severe Allergic Reactions to Insect Stings, p. 75.)

SYMPTOMS

Insect stings can cause any or all of the following symptoms, which occur at the bite area and may last 48 to 72 hours:

- Pain
- Swelling
- Redness
- Itching
- Burning

WHAT TO DO

1. If the insect has left its stinger behind, carefully remove it by gently scraping the skin with a dull knife blade, card edge, or fingernail. *Do not* squeeze it with tweezers, as this may cause more venom to enter the body.
2. Wash the area with soap and water. Do not break blisters caused by fire ants. Doing so could cause an infection.
3. Place ice wrapped in cloth or cold compresses on the sting area to decrease the absorption and spread of the venom.
4. Take an oral antihistamine to help ease the symptoms.

Avoiding Bee Stings

Here are some steps you can take to avoid bee stings:

- Don't disturb nests.
- Clean up food spills and remove garbage frequently.
- Eliminate hives by spraying insecticide in them at night when it's dark and the bees are inside the hives and quiet.

Multiple Stings

Sometimes, when a person receives several insect stings, he or she may have a reaction that is not necessarily life-threatening, but still requires an evaluation by a doctor.

Multiple insect stings can cause any or all of the following symptoms:

- Rapid onset of swelling
- Headache
- Muscle cramps
- Fever
- Drowsiness

1. If the insects have left stingers behind, carefully remove them by gently scraping the skin with a dull knife blade, a credit card edge, or a fingernail. *Do not* squeeze the stingers with tweezers, because this can cause more venom to enter the body.
2. Wash the sting sites with soap and water.
3. Place ice wrapped in cloth or cold compresses on sting sites.
4. Take an oral antihistamine to help ease symptoms.
5. Seek medical attention, as other medication may be needed.

Severe Allergic Reactions to Insect Stings

An allergic reaction to insect stings can be life-threatening and can result from one or more bites or stings. Allergic reactions often occur in people who have been bitten or stung previously and have become sensitized to the particular venom.

Anaphylactic shock, which can occur from such stings, is a total body allergic reaction. Anyone who knows he or she is allergic to bee venom should always carry an anaphylaxis emergency kit and wear a medical identification tag.

Anaphylactic shock can cause any or all of the following symptoms:

- Severe swelling in other parts of the body such as the eyes, lips, and tongue, as well as at the bite site
- Hives or hivelike rash on the body
- Coughing or wheezing
- Severe itching
- Difficulty breathing
- Stomach cramps

INJURIES AND ILLNESSES

- Nausea and vomiting
- Anxiety
- Weakness
- Dizziness
- Bluish tinge to the skin
- Collapse
- Unconsciousness

WHAT TO DO

If an emergency kit for insect stings is not available:

1. Call 911 (or your local emergency number), or take the person to the nearest hospital emergency department immediately.
2. If the person is not breathing, maintain an open airway. Restore breathing and circulation, if necessary. (See pp. 31–50.)

If an emergency kit for insect stings is available:

1. If the victim is unable to administer an injection of adrenaline, give the injection, carefully following the instructions in the emergency kit.
2. Seek medical attention immediately. Call 911 (or your local emergency number) or take the victim to the nearest hospital emergency department.

SPIDER AND TICK BITES

Black Widow Spider Bites

Black widow spider bites are particularly harmful to very young children, the elderly, and the chronically ill. The spiders appear most often during the summer months, usually in garages, barns, and garbage heaps. Their webs have an irregular shape, unlike most other spider webs.

SYMPTOMS

The bite of a black widow spider can cause any or all of the following symptoms:

- Slight redness and swelling around the bite
- Sharp pain around the bite

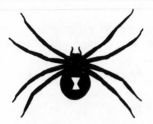

BLACK WIDOW SPIDER

The black widow spider has a shiny black body less than 1 inch in length. Its unique feature is a red hourglass marking on the underside of its body.

- Profuse sweating
- Nausea and vomiting
- Stomach cramps or hard, rigid abdomen within 1 hour of the bite
- Possible muscle cramps in other parts of the body
- Tightness in the chest and difficulty breathing and talking
- Weakness
- Swelling of the face

WHAT TO DO

If the person is not breathing:
1. Call 911 (or your local emergency number) or take the person to the nearest hospital emergency department.
2. Maintain an open airway. Restore breathing and circulation if necessary. (See pp. 31–50.)

If the person is breathing:
1. Keep the bitten area lower than the victim's heart.
2. Place ice wrapped in cloth or cold compresses on the bitten area.
3. Keep the victim quiet.
4. Seek medical attention promptly, preferably at the nearest hospital emergency department. If you can catch the spider safely, take it with you.

INJURIES AND ILLNESSES

77

Brown Recluse Spider Bites

Brown recluse spiders are found from spring to fall, usually in at-
tics, closets, storage sheds, woodpiles, or vacant buildings, or
under rocks. They are especially active at night and people often
get bites while sleeping on sheets that have been in long-term
storage. Brown recluse spider bites are particularly harmful to
very young children and older people, causing severe, deep, irre-
versible tissue damage around the bite area. Immediate medical
attention is required.

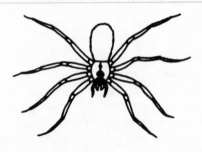

BROWN RECLUSE SPIDER

The brown recluse spider (also called the fiddleback or violin spider) is
characterized by a dark brown violin-shaped marking on the top front
portion of its body.

SYMPTOMS

The bite of a brown recluse spider can cause any or all of the following symptoms:

- A stinging sensation at the time of the bite
- Redness at the site of the bite, which later disappears as a
  blister forms
- Pain that may become more severe over the next 8 hours
- Chills, fever, nausea, vomiting, joint pains, and rash over the
  next 48 hours
- Destruction of tissue that may form an open ulcer that could
  persist for months
- Blood in urine within 1 day of bite

WHAT TO DO

Follow steps in What to Do under Black Widow Spider Bites, p. 77.

> ### WARNING
>
> **LIFE-THREATENING SYMPTOMS**
>
> If a person who has been bitten by a brown recluse spider develops the following symptoms within 48 hours, take him or her immediately to the nearest hospital emergency department:
>
> • Fever
> • Blood in urine
> • Rash
> • Joint pain

Tarantula Bites

Tarantula bites are not usually as serious as those of the black widow spider or the brown recluse spider. Tarantulas are usually between 1 and 3 inches long and tend to move more slowly than other spiders.

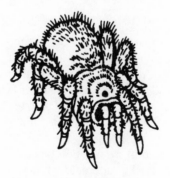

TARANTULA
The tarantula is a large spider with a very hairy body and legs.

INJURIES AND ILLNESSES

SYMPTOMS

The bite of a tarantula may cause any or all of the following symptoms:

- Severe itching
- Mild pain at the time of the bite
- A severe, painful wound a few days after the bite

WHAT TO DO

1. Pull off spider hairs with adhesive or cellophane tape.
2. Wash the area with soap and water.
3. Place ice wrapped in cloth or cold compresses on the bite area.
4. Elevate the affected part of the body above the level of the heart.
5. To relieve discomfort, take an antihistamine and/or a pain reliever such as ibuprofen, naproxen, or acetaminophen as directed.
6. If the person has shortness of breath, weakness, or chest pain, or if he or she faints, call 911 (or your local emergency number) or take him or her to the nearest hospital emergency department.

Tick Bites

Ticks are arachnids that thrive in wooded and grassy areas and feed on animals such as deer, mice, and rabbits. Ticks can transmit disease-causing organisms from animals to people. People who live near wooded and grassy areas or who camp or hike near them are most susceptible to tick bites. Family pets can transport ticks into the home. The worst time of the year for tick infestation is May through August. Because of the risk of developing a serious infection from a tick bite—especially Lyme disease (see p. 82) or Rocky Mountain spotted fever (see p. 83)—you should always see your doctor for an evaluation if you have been bitten by a tick or even suspect that you have been bitten by one. Your doctor will probably give you a blood test to determine if you have an infection. If the initial blood test is negative, as it often is in the early stages of infection, your doctor may ask you to return for additional blood tests. Both Lyme disease and Rocky Mountain spotted fever can be treated successfully with antibiotics in the early stages.

Normal-size tick   Tick engorged with blood

TICKS

Ticks are tiny, about ⅛ inch in length. When biting a person or animal, a tick attaches itself to the skin with its mouth and, engorged with blood, expands to five to seven times its original size.

WHAT TO DO

To remove a tick from the skin:
1. Do not touch the tick with your fingers; put on a pair of rubber gloves if you have them or protect your fingers with a tissue. Do not use a match or lighted cigarette on the tick because doing so could cause the tick to embed itself farther in the skin.
2. To remove a tick, use tweezers to grasp the tick's head and mouth as close to the skin as possible (but being careful not to crush or twist the tick's body). Pull the tick out gently but firmly and steadily in one piece. If the tick's head breaks off from the body, it could become embedded in the skin.
3. Dispose of the tick by flushing it down the toilet or placing it in a jar of alcohol.
4. Wash your hands thoroughly with soap and water.
5. Clean the wound with an antiseptic such as rubbing alcohol.
6. See a doctor to determine proper treatment and to make sure the tick's whole body has been removed.

If the tick becomes embedded in the skin:
1. Pinch the outer layer of skin that contains the embedded head and mouth of the tick and carefully scrape it (do not cut it) with a sharp, sterilized single-edge razor blade.
2. Clean the wound with an antiseptic such as rubbing alcohol.

3. If you don't want to remove the tick's head yourself, see a physician. You should see a physician anyway after removing a tick to make sure you have removed all of it.

Avoiding Tick Bites

The following steps can help you avoid tick bites when you're in an area that could be infested with ticks:

- At home, mow your lawn regularly; clear out brush and leaf litter; stack woodpiles neatly in a dry location, preferably off the ground; remove leaves and the remains of plants from the garden in the fall.
- Always wear shoes or boots and socks, long pants with socks over the bottom of the pants, and a long-sleeved shirt tucked into the pants when camping or hiking.
- Wear light-colored clothing with a tight weave so you can see the ticks more easily and avoid skin contact.
- Check all parts of your body and your clothes for ticks twice a day and brush yourself and your companions with a broom or towel after hiking.
- Keep long hair pulled back; comb or brush your hair after hiking.
- Shower and shampoo your hair after leaving a tick-infested area, if possible, and wash and dry your clothes to eliminate any unseen ticks.
- Keep towels and clothing off the ground at camping areas and at the beach.
- Walk only on marked, clear, well-worn trails whenever possible.
- Use an insect repellent with chemicals formulated to ward off ticks (such as N,N-diethyl-meta-toluamide or permethrin).
- Check with your veterinarian for sprays or powders to use on pets.

Lyme Disease

Lyme disease, named for its discovery in Old Lyme, Connecticut, is a bacterial infection transmitted by the bite of a tick. The tick that can carry Lyme disease thrives in wooded and grassy areas throughout the United States and acquires the bacteria by feeding on infected deer and mice.

Although Lyme disease is not life-threatening, it can be debilitating. In untreated cases, the disease can lead to heart irregularities, muscle weakness or numbness in the face and limbs, sensitivity to touch, arthritis, and meningitis (inflammation of the membranes that cover the brain and spinal cord).

SYMPTOMS

Symptoms of meningitis include severe headaches, lethargy, and a stiff neck. If you notice these symptoms or any or all of the following symptoms of Lyme disease (some of which may not appear for several days or months after the tick bite), seek medical attention immediately:

- A round, red, expanding rash or blotch at the site of the bite within 3 to 30 days after the bite (not everyone develops a rash). As the rash expands, the central part may appear pale and the border deep red, resembling a bull's-eye. The area is about 6 inches in diameter and usually appears on the thigh or groin or near the armpit, not necessarily at the site of the bite. The rash may persist for 3 to 5 weeks.
- Fever
- Chills
- Headache
- Stiff neck
- Fatigue
- Muscle and joint pain
- Dizziness
- Memory disturbance
- Red eyes

Rocky Mountain Spotted Fever

Rocky Mountain spotted fever is a serious but rare infection transmitted by the bite of a tick. Although first recognized in the Rocky Mountains, the disease can occur anywhere in the United States and in Canada. The infection is caused by a parasitic microorganism called a rickettsia. The tick feeds on small mammals, such as rabbits and rodents, and can then transmit the rickettsia from the animals to people. If you notice any of the symptoms listed below, seek medical attention immediately.

INJURIES AND ILLNESSES

Rocky Mountain spotted fever can cause any or all of the following symptoms, which may appear suddenly or not appear for several weeks after the bite:

- Headache
- Fever (usually high)
- Loss of appetite
- Nausea and/or vomiting
- Rash (pink to deep red spots) that appears first (within 2 to 5 days after the bite) on the wrists and ankles and then spreads to the palms of the hands, the soles of the feet, the forearms, and eventually the rest of the body
- Swelling of the inner eyelids and around the eyes
- Swelling of the feet and hands

MARINE LIFE STINGS

Stings from certain types of marine life are poisonous. Four of the most common offenders are the Portuguese man-of-war, the jellyfish, the scorpionfish, and the stingray.

Portuguese Man-of-War and Jellyfish

Jellyfish can be poisonous even when they're dead because they still contain active stinging cells. The Portuguese man-of-war is usually found in the Gulf of Mexico in late summer; the jellyfish can be found in the Florida area, the Chesapeake Bay area, and in the South Pacific.

SYMPTOMS

Stings from the Portuguese man-of-war and the jellyfish can cause any or all of the following symptoms:

- Intense burning pain
- Reddening of the skin
- Skin rash
- Muscle cramps
- Nausea and vomiting
- Difficulty breathing

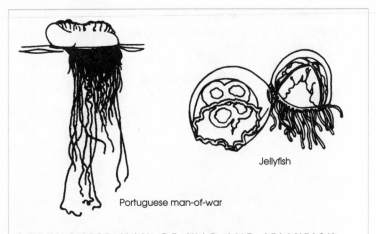

PORTUGUESE MAN-OF-WAR AND JELLYFISH
Stings from the Portuguese man-of-war and the jellyfish are poisonous.

INJURIES AND ILLNESSES

> **WARNING**
>
> SEVERE MARINE LIFE STINGS
>
> If a sting affects more than half of an arm or leg or if the victim is unconscious, call 911 (or your local emergency number) or transport the victim immediately to the nearest hospital emergency department.

WHAT TO DO

If stung by a Portuguese man-of-war:
Wrap cloth around your hands (or use tweezers, pliers, or forceps) and carefully remove any attached tentacles. *An unattached tentacle can still sting.* Then continue with steps 1 through 4 below.

If stung by a Portuguese man-of-war or a jellyfish:
1. Wash the affected area with seawater or vinegar (3- to 5-percent acetic acid) to deactivate the stinging cells. Do not use fresh water (or tap water) because fresh water can stimulate the stinging cells to release venom.

2. To help remove the stinging cells that are still attached to the skin, apply shaving cream and gently shave the area or rub with a paste of sand or mud and seawater.

3. To relieve discomfort, apply a mild hydrocortisone cream to the area or take an oral antihistamine.

4. If the person has shortness of breath, weakness, or chest pain, or if he or she faints, call 911 (or your local emergency number) or take the person to the nearest hospital emergency department.

Stingrays and Scorpionfish

Stingrays (also called devilfish) are flat fish that inhabit the bottom of shallow tropical waters. Scorpionfish, which also inhabit the bottom of shallow tropical waters, are colorful fish that are found throughout the world. Scorpionfish include lionfish, butterfly cod, bullroot, and stonefish.

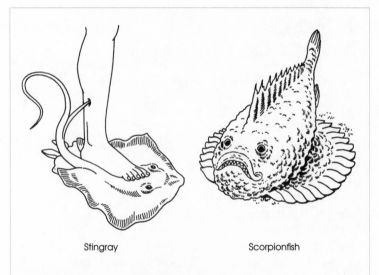

Stingray   Scorpionfish

STINGRAYS AND SCORPIONFISH
When disturbed, which usually means being stepped on, a stingray will whip its tail to inject venom, usually into the person's leg. The spine on a stingray's tail can penetrate a rubber or leather boot or wet suit. Scorpionfish use the spines on their back as stinging agents. Scorpionfish can appear to be dead when they are not.

Stings from the stingray or scorpionfish can cause any or all of the following symptoms:

- Intense pain in the area of the sting
- Nausea, vomiting, and/or abdominal cramps
- Fast heart rate
- Dizziness
- Muscle cramps or spasms

WHAT TO DO

1. Have the victim immerse the affected area in a container of hot but not scalding (113°F) water and take him or her to the nearest hospital emergency department. The victim should keep the area immersed in the water during transport because it takes about 30 to 90 minutes to deactivate the fish venom.
2. If possible, keep the affected area immobilized.
3. If you cannot get the victim to a hospital emergency department immediately, have him or her immerse the affected area in hot water for at least 90 minutes and seek medical attention as soon as possible.

SCORPION STINGS

Some species of scorpions are more poisonous than others. Scorpion stings are particularly harmful to very young children. Scorpions, which tend to hide under wood or in crevices, are usually found in desert areas of the southwestern United States, Mexico, and Brazil. They are most active during hot weather and at night.

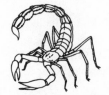

SCORPION
The scorpion looks like a 2-inch-long lobster or crab. It has a set of pincers and a stinger located in the tail, which arches over its back.

INJURIES AND ILLNESSES

SYMPTOMS

A scorpion sting may cause any or all of the following symptoms:

- Severe burning pain at the site of the sting
- Nausea and vomiting
- Stomach pain
- Numbness and tingling in the affected area
- Spasm of jaw muscles, making opening of the mouth difficult
- Fast heart rate
- Blurred vision
- Twitching and spasm of affected muscles
- Convulsions
- Coma

WHAT TO DO

If the victim is not breathing:
1. Call 911 (or your local emergency number).
2. Maintain an open airway. Restore breathing and circulation if necessary. (See pp. 31–50.)

If the victim is breathing:
1. Keep the bitten area lower than the victim's heart.
2. Place ice wrapped in cloth or cold compresses on the bitten area.
3. Keep the victim quiet.
4. Seek medical attention promptly, preferably at the nearest hospital emergency department.

Avoiding Scorpion Bites

Here are some steps you can take to avoid scorpion bites:

- Remove all wood debris, including dead wood and firewood, from around your home.
- Set up your campsite away from wood debris.
- Always wear footwear in scorpion-infested areas.
- When camping, shake out clothing and sheets before you use them.

SNAKEBITES

When you are bitten by a snake, it is important to know whether or not it is poisonous. Poisonous snakes in the United States include the rattlesnake, cottonmouth (water moccasin), copperhead, and coral snake. Rattlesnakes can be found all over the country and are responsible for two out of three poisonous snakebites in the United States. Cottonmouth and copperhead snakes are found primarily in the southeast and south central parts of the United States. Coral snakes are found primarily in the southeast. Snakebites are most common during the summer months and usually affect the arms or legs.

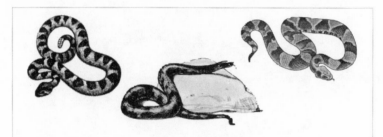

RATTLESNAKE, COTTONMOUTH, AND COPPERHEAD

The rattlesnake (*left*), cottonmouth (*center*), and copperhead (*right*) have deep poison pits between their nostrils and eyes, slitlike eyes, and two long fangs. A unique feature of the rattlesnake is the set of rattles at the end of the tail. A distinctive feature of the cottonmouth (also called a water moccasin) is the white coloring inside the mouth. Unique features of the copperhead are a copper-colored head and a pinkish-gray body with a brown hourglass pattern.

Poisonous Snakes

The rattlesnake, cottonmouth, and copperhead have a triangular-shaped head and deep pits (poison sacs) between the nostrils and the eyes. They also have slitlike eyes rather than the round eyes of nonpoisonous snakes. The coral snake is an exception—instead of the slitlike eyes of the other poisonous snakes, it has round eyes. Poisonous snakes also have long fangs that leave distinctive marks followed by a row of tooth marks. Most nonpoi-

89

sonous snakes, by contrast, have rounded heads and round eyes. They do not have pits between their eyes and nostrils and they do not have fangs.

The coral snake is a member of the cobra family. It has red, yellow, and black rings. The yellow rings are narrow and *always* separate the red rings from the black. A rhyme to remember that identifies the coral snake is "Red on yellow will kill a fellow, red on black won't hurt Jack." The coral snake is smaller than the pit vipers, has round eyes like nonpoisonous snakes, and *always* has a black nose. Its venom is highly toxic to humans. Unlike the other poisonous snakes, which usually bite once and let go, the coral snake hangs on and chews the victim's flesh.

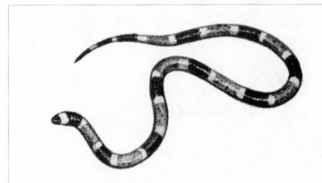

CORAL SNAKE
Unlike the rattlesnake, copperhead, and cottonmouth, the coral snake has round, rather than slitlike, eyes. It has fangs like the other poisonous snakes. Its markings consist of yellow, red, and black rings, with the narrow yellow rings always separating the red rings from the black. The coral snake always has a black nose and is about 2 to 4 feet long.

If you can do so safely, try to capture and kill the snake without deforming its head and take it with you to the medical facility. However, keep in mind that the severed head of a snake can contain poison for up to 1 hour after the snake has died, so handle it carefully. If it is not possible to capture the snake, remember its characteristics. You might be able to capture it later because, even several hours later, most snakes can be found within 20 feet of where they were when they bit a person.

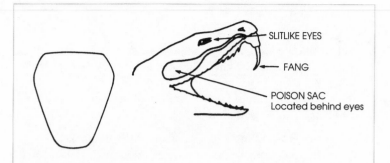

CHARACTERISTICS OF SOME POISONOUS SNAKES

Most poisonous snakes have a triangular-shaped head (left), oval or slit-like eyes, deep pits (poison sacs) between their nostrils and eyes, and fangs (right). The rattlesnake, copperhead, and cottonmouth all share these characteristics. The coral snake is an exception because it has round eyes.

Rattlesnake, Cottonmouth, or Copperhead Bites

If there is no swelling within 4 hours of a snakebite, the snake was probably not poisonous, but you should still seek medical attention. Bites from a rattlesnake, cottonmouth, or copperhead can cause any or all of the following symptoms:

SYMPTOMS

- Severe pain
- Rapid swelling
- Discoloration of the skin around the bite
- Weakness
- Nausea and vomiting
- Difficulty breathing
- Blurred vision
- Convulsions
- Numbness in arms or legs
- Redness at site of bite

If the person is not breathing:

1. Call 911 (or your local emergency number) or transport the person immediately to the nearest hospital emergency department.
2. Maintain an open airway. Restore breathing and circulation if necessary. (See pp. 31–50.)

If the person is breathing and a snakebite kit is available:

1. Place suction cups from the kit over the wound and draw out body fluids containing venom. This measure is most effective when used within minutes of the snakebite. Carefully follow the instructions in the kit.
2. Keep the victim quiet to slow circulation, which will help stop the spread of the venom.
3. Remove rings, watches, and other jewelry.
4. Wash the bite area thoroughly with soap and water. Do not apply ice water or ice; it could damage the tissue.
5. Cover the wound with a sterile or clean bandage.
6. Immobilize a bitten arm or leg with a splint or other suitable device and keep it just below the level of the heart. *Do not* let the victim walk unless absolutely necessary, and then slowly.
7. Give the victim small sips of water if desired and if he or she has no difficulty swallowing. *Do not* give water if the victim is nauseated, vomiting, having convulsions, or unconscious. *Do not* give the victim alcoholic beverages.
8. Seek medical attention promptly, preferably at the nearest hospital emergency department. If possible, have someone telephone ahead to tell of the poisonous snakebite and type of snake so that antivenom serum can be readied.

Coral Snake Bites

SYMPTOMS

Symptoms from a coral snakebite, which may not occur for up to 6 hours after the bite, may include any or all of the following:

- Slight pain and swelling at the site of the bite
- Blurred vision
- Drooping eyelids

- Difficulty speaking or swallowing
- Heavy drooling
- Drowsiness
- Heavy sweating
- Nausea and vomiting
- Difficulty breathing
- Paralysis
- Pain in joints
- Confusion
- Weakness
- Dizziness
- Slurred speech

WHAT TO DO

If the person is not breathing:

1. Call 911 (or your local emergency number) or transport the person immediately to the nearest hospital emergency department.
2. Maintain an open airway. Restore breathing and circulation if necessary. (See pp. 31–50.)

If the person is breathing and a snakebite kit is available:

1. Place suction cups from the kit over the wound and draw out body fluids containing venom. This measure is most effective when used within minutes of the snakebite. Carefully follow the instructions in the kit.
2. Keep the victim quiet to slow circulation, which will help stop the spread of the venom.
3. Remove rings, watches, and other jewelry.
4. Wash the bite area thoroughly with soap and water. Do not apply ice water or ice; it could damage the tissue.
5. Cover the wound with a sterile or clean bandage.
6. Immobilize a bitten arm or leg with a splint or other suitable device and keep it just below the level of the heart. *Do not* let the victim walk unless absolutely necessary, and then slowly.
7. Give the victim small sips of water if desired and if he or she has no difficulty swallowing. *Do not* give water if the victim is nauseated, vomiting, having convulsions, or unconscious. *Do not* give the victim alcoholic beverages.
8. Seek medical attention promptly, preferably at the nearest hospital emergency department. If possible, have someone tele-

INJURIES AND ILLNESSES

phone ahead to tell of the poisonous snakebite and type of snake so that antivenom serum can be readied.

Nonpoisonous Snakes

SYMPTOMS

Bites from nonpoisonous snakes can cause any or all of the following symptoms:

- Pain
- Swelling
- Mild bleeding

WHAT TO DO

1. Keep the affected area below the level of the victim's heart.
2. Remove all rings, watches, and other jewelry.
3. Clean the area thoroughly with soap and water. Do not apply ice or ice water to the bite.
4. Put a bandage or clean cloth over the wound.
5. Seek medical attention. Medication or a tetanus shot may be necessary.

POISONOUS LIZARD BITES

The Gila monster and the Mexican beaded lizard are the only poisonous lizards found in North America, usually in southern Arizona and northwestern Mexico. Both of these lizards are longer than 1 foot and have heavy bodies with a beadlike surface, flat heads, short legs, and round, thick tails. The Gila monster's skin is patterned in pink or orange and black; the Mexican beaded lizard's skin is dark purple and black. Although poisonous, their bites are rarely fatal. The Gila monster hangs on tenaciously when it bites and must be removed carefully to prevent the teeth from remaining embedded in the skin.

SYMPTOMS

Bites from a Gila monster or Mexican beaded lizard can cause any or all of the following symptoms:

- Immediate, intense pain that shoots up from the site of the bite (usually the arm or leg)
- Swelling at the site of the bite
- Blueness of the skin at the site of the bite
- Nausea and/or vomiting
- Fainting
- Weakness
- Sweating
- Fever and chills
- High blood pressure

WHAT TO DO

If you are being bitten by a Gila monster and it is holding on by its teeth:

Try to remove it without breaking its teeth by quickly and carefully submerging the affected area of your body (and the lizard) in cold water. If this doesn't release the lizard's hold, place a strong stick between the bitten area and the back of the lizard's mouth and push the stick against the rear of the lizard's jaw. Do not try to remove any teeth that are still embedded in the skin; a doctor will need to remove them. Once the lizard lets go, continue with steps 1 through 4 below.

For a bite by either a Gila monster or a Mexican beaded lizard:

1. Wash the wound thoroughly with soap and water and rinse it under running water for 10 to 20 minutes.
2. Cover the wound with a clean dressing and apply pressure for 5 minutes if the wound is bleeding.
3. Immobilize the affected limb at heart level.
4. Seek medical attention immediately.

See Also: Shock (Anaphylactic Shock), p. 240; Unconsciousness, p. 259.

INJURIES AND ILLNESSES

Blood may flow from a vein or an artery or both. Blood from veins is dark red and flows steadily. Blood from arteries is bright red and usually spurts from the wound. Bleeding from an artery is more critical than bleeding from a vein because blood is being pumped out at a faster rate, leading to greater blood loss. Severe bleeding from an artery can be fatal. If you notice that blood is spurting from a wound, call 911 (or your local emergency number) or take the person to a hospital emergency department or doctor's office immediately.*

EXTERNAL BLEEDING

WHAT TO DO

Direct Pressure

Direct pressure is the preferred treatment in bleeding injuries and, though it may cause some pain, constant pressure is usually all that is necessary to stop the bleeding.

Direct Pressure for Bleeding

To apply direct pressure:

1. Place a thick clean compress (sterile gauze or a soft clean cloth such as a handkerchief, towel, undershirt, or strips from a

*NOTE: There is concern among those who provide first aid—even on a one-time basis—that HIV (the virus that causes AIDS) may be contracted from a victim's body fluids. It is extremely unlikely that you will contract HIV from the blood or saliva of a person who requires mouth-to-mouth resuscitation or CPR. HIV can be passed to others through an infected person's blood and semen. The virus may be present in saliva, but cases in which it has been transmitted through saliva are unknown at present. People who regularly come in contact with blood or saliva—doctors, paramedics, other emergency department personnel, and dentists—wear protective clothing including face masks and gloves. Even among these health-care professionals, the risk of contracting HIV is extremely low.

sheet) directly over the
entire wound and press
firmly with the palm of
your hand. (If cloth is not
available, use bare hands
or fingers, but they
should be as clean as
possible.)

2. Continue to apply steady
   pressure. A limb that is
   bleeding severely should
   be raised above the level
   of the victim's heart.

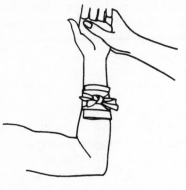

3. *Do not* disturb any blood clots that form on the compress. If
   blood soaks through the compress, leave the compress in
   place and apply another compress over it. Continue applying
   pressure, using firmer hand pressure over a wider area.

4. If bleeding stops or slows, apply a pressure bandage to hold
   the compress snugly in place. To apply a pressure bandage,
   place the center of the gauze, cloth strips, or necktie directly
   over the compress. Pull steadily while wrapping both ends
   around the injury. Tie a knot over the compress. *Do not* wrap
   the bandage so tightly
   that it cuts off arterial circulation. (Arteries carry
   blood away from the
   heart to the extremities.)
   A pulse can be felt on an
   artery. You should feel a
   pulse *below* the bandage,
   meaning at a point on an
   artery that is farthest
   away from the trunk of
   the body.

5. Keep an injured limb
   elevated.

NOTE: You can stop bleeding in the mouth by placing a sterile
gauze pad over the wound and applying pressure with your hand
or by biting on it, depending on where the bleeding is.

Pressure Points

Applying pressure to pressure points (see illustration on p. 99) should be done *only* if bleeding does not stop after elevating an injured limb and applying direct pressure to the wound itself. This technique is used to press the artery supplying blood to the wound against the underlying bone and cut off circulation to the affected area. Applying pressure to pressure points is used in conjunction with applying direct pressure to a wound and elevating the wound above the heart. However, before using this technique, call 911 (or your local emergency number) for immediate medical help. Severe blood loss can be fatal.

To stop severe bleeding from an arm:
1. Grasp the victim's arm bone midway between the armpit and the elbow with your thumb on the outside of the arm and the flat surface of your fingers on the inside of the arm, where you may actually feel the artery pulsating.
2. Squeeze your fingers firmly toward your thumb against the arm bone until the bleeding stops.

To stop severe bleeding from a leg:
1. Lay the victim on his or her back, if possible.
2. Place the heel of your hand on the front center part of the victim's thigh at the crease of the groin and press down firmly. *Do not* continue pressing any longer than necessary to stop the bleeding. However, if bleeding recurs after you remove your hand, reapply pressure.

Tourniquet

Use a tourniquet only in life-threatening situations, when severe bleeding in an arm or leg cannot be stopped by direct pressure on the wound or by direct pressure on a pressure point. In emergencies, such as partial or complete amputation, in which the victim is in danger of bleeding to death, the risk of losing a limb is secondary to saving his or her life. Before applying a tourniquet, call 911 (or your local emergency number) for immediate medical attention.

To apply a tourniquet:
1. Find a strip of cloth, belt, tie, scarf, or other flat material that is 2 or more inches wide and long enough to wrap around the limb twice, with ends for tying.

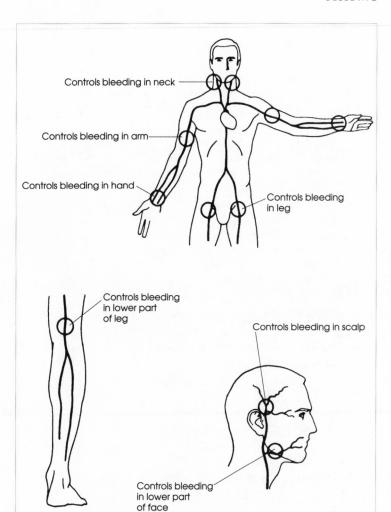

Controls bleeding in neck

Controls bleeding in arm

Controls bleeding in hand

Controls bleeding
in leg

Controls bleeding
in lower part
of leg

Controls bleeding in scalp

Controls bleeding
in lower part
of face

INJURIES AND ILLNESSES

PRESSURE POINTS ON THE BODY

For severe bleeding that cannot be controlled by applying direct pressure to the wound, pressing the artery that supplies blood to the wound firmly against the underlying bone can help. Apply pressure only until the bleeding stops. The circled areas on the arteries show the places to apply pressure to control bleeding in specific injured areas of the body. Each artery has a corresponding artery with a corresponding pressure point on the other side of the body.

2. Place the tourniquet just above the wound (between the wound and the body) but not touching the wound. Wrap it twice around the limb and tie a half knot.
3. Place a stick, pen, or other strong, straight object on top of the half knot and tie two full knots over the stick.
4. Twist the stick to tighten the tourniquet until the bleeding stops.
5. Tie the loose ends of the tourniquet around the stick to hold it in place. Another method of securing the stick is to tie a second strip of cloth or other material around the free end of the stick and tie the cloth around the limb. *Do not* loosen or remove the tourniquet once it has been applied and do not cover it.
6. Attach a note to the victim's clothing stating the time the tourniquet was applied.

INTERNAL BLEEDING

Internal bleeding is not always obvious. You may suspect internal bleeding if the victim has been in an accident, fallen, or received a severe body blow. Internal bleeding in the chest, abdomen, or thigh can be life-threatening.

SYMPTOMS

Internal bleeding can cause any or all of the following symptoms:

- Vomit that resembles coffee grounds or is red
- Coughed-up blood that is bright red and/or frothy (bubbly)
- Stools that are black or contain bright red blood
- Paleness
- Cold, clammy skin
- Rapid and weak pulse
- Light-headedness
- Distended (swollen) abdomen
- Restlessness
- Thirst
- Apprehension
- Mental confusion

WHAT TO DO

1. Call 911 (or your local emergency number) or transport the person immediately to the nearest hospital emergency department.
2. If the person is not breathing, maintain an open airway. Restore breathing and circulation if necessary. (See pp. 31–50.)
3. *Do not* give the victim anything to drink.
4. Calm and reassure the victim.

See Also: Amputations, p. 68; Pregnancy Danger Signs, p. 228; Shock (Shock From Severe Injury), p. 241; Wounds, p. 264.

INJURIES AND ILLNESSES

Blisters are usually caused by clothing (such as shoes) or equipment repeatedly rubbing against the skin. In general, the best way to handle blisters is to leave them alone. They usually heal on their own.

WHAT TO DO

If the blister is small and unopened and will receive no further irritation:
Cover it with a sterile gauze pad and bandage in place. The fluid in the blister will eventually be absorbed by the skin and it will heal itself.

If the blister accidentally breaks, exposing raw skin:
Wash the area gently with soap and water and cover with a sterile bandage. The skin will regrow its outer layers.

If the blister is large and likely to be broken by routine activity:
Seek medical attention for treatment.

If medical attention is not readily available:
1. Gently clean the area with soap and water. Sterilize a needle by holding it over an open flame. Puncture the lower edge of the blister with the needle. Press the blister gently to force out fluid. Cover the area with a sterile bandage.
2. Always look for signs of infection such as redness, pus, or red streaks leading from the wound. Seek medical attention promptly if these symptoms appear.

See Also: Bleeding, p. 96.

BREATHING PROBLEMS
IN CHILDREN

Breathing problems in infants and young children are common and usually are not serious. However, in some instances, a serious condition does arise that requires immediate medical attention.

CROUP

Croup is a group of symptoms arising from various respiratory conditions that occur most frequently in children under 3. Croup is generally caused by a virus, a bacterial infection, or an allergy. Its symptoms occur most often in fall and winter.

Most attacks of croup occur at night after a child has gone to bed. Often the child has had a mild cold before the attack. Croup that occurs during the day generally becomes more severe in the evening.

SYMPTOMS

Croup can cause any or all of the following symptoms:

• Difficulty breathing, particularly inhaling
• Croaking sound upon inhaling (stridor)
• Hoarseness
• Hacking, barklike cough
• Bluish tinge to the skin and lips when the attack is severe
• Restlessness

WHAT TO DO

1. Reassure the child so that he or she does not become overly frightened.
2. *Do not* place a spoon or other object in the child's mouth. This will not aid breathing and may cause airway obstruction.

3. To help the child breathe, place a cool-mist vaporizer in the child's room. Or sit with the child in a closed, steam-filled bathroom. (To create steam, let hot water run from the shower or tub for several minutes with the bathroom door closed.) *Do not* put the child in the water. Remain in the bathroom for 20 to 30 minutes. A small child can be held up high where the steam accumulates.

4. Call 911 (or your local emergency number) or take the child immediately to the nearest hospital emergency department if symptoms continue and one or more of the following happens:

- Condition worsens after the child has been awake a short while
- Extreme difficulty breathing
- Croaking sound (stridor) while inhaling, even when the child is calm
- Blue skin and lips
- Sudden moderate fever or high fever
- Becomes agitated or appears exhausted and incapacitated

WARNING

BLOCKED WINDPIPE

If the child begins to drool, which may indicate a life-threatening condition called epiglottitis (see below), seek medical attention promptly. Call 911 (or your local emergency number) or take the child immediately to the nearest hospital emergency department. *Keep the child in a sitting position.*

EPIGLOTTITIS

Epiglottitis is a life-threatening medical condition in which the epiglottis—the flap of tissue at the back of the throat that closes off the windpipe (trachea) during swallowing—becomes infected, inflamed, and swollen, partially closing off the airway. It usually occurs in children between the ages of 2 and 7. Symptoms may appear after the child has had a severe sore throat or cold.

A child with any of these symptoms should be treated by paramedics or taken *without delay* to a hospital emergency department:

- Difficulty swallowing
- Drooling
- Little or no voice
- Sits straight up with jaw thrust forward in an attempt to keep the airway open
- Fever

WHAT TO DO

- Call 911 (or your local emergency number) or take the child *without delay* to a hospital emergency department. *Keep the child in a sitting position.*
- *Do not* place a spoon or other object in the child's mouth. This will not aid breathing and may cause airway obstruction.
- Do not agitate the child.

SUDDEN INFANT DEATH SYNDROME

Sudden infant death syndrome (SIDS) is the death of an apparently healthy infant under 1 year (usually 6 months or younger) for which no cause can be found. SIDS occurs most frequently during the winter months.

WHAT TO DO

1. Call 911 (or your local emergency number).
2. Attempt to restore breathing and circulation. (See pp. 31–50.)

Preventing SIDS

Here are some steps you can take to reduce your baby's risk of SIDS:

- Always put your infant to sleep on his or her back.
- Make sure the crib mattress is firm and flat.

INJURIES AND ILLNESSES

- Never put your baby to sleep on a beanbag chair or waterbed.
- Do not place soft, fluffy toys, pillows, blankets, comforters, or sheepskins in the crib.
- Do not let your child get overheated while sleeping—remove any unnecessary coverings from the crib and don't swaddle or overdress him or her.
- Never use plastic sheets.
- Do not allow smoking in or near your child's sleeping area.

A break or crack in a bone is a fracture. A fracture may be closed or open. In a closed fracture, the broken bone does not come through the skin. Usually the skin is not broken near the fracture site.

In an open fracture, there is an open wound that extends down to the bone, or parts of the broken bone may stick out through the skin. An open break is usually more serious because of severe bleeding and the greater possibility of infection.

Always suspect a broken neck or spinal injury if the victim is unconscious or has a head injury, neck pain, tingling, or paralysis in the arms or legs. (See Head, Neck, and Back Injuries, p. 194.)

Do not move the victim, particularly if he or she has head, neck, or spine injuries (or if paramedics or other trained ambulance personnel are readily available), unless the victim is in immediate danger from a fire, explosion, traffic, or other life-threatening situation. If the victim must be moved, immobilize the injured part first. For example, tie the injured leg to the uninjured leg, if possible.

Do not lift a victim with a suspected neck or spinal injury out of the water without a back support, such as a board. If the victim must be dragged to safety, *do not* drag him or her sideways but pull by the armpits or legs in the direction of the length of the body, *keeping the head in line with the body. Do not* let the victim's body bend or twist, particularly the neck or back. (See Head, Neck, and Back Injuries, p. 194.)

SYMPTOMS

Always suspect a broken bone under any of the following circumstances:

- The victim felt or heard a bone snap.
- The site of the injury is painful or tender, particularly when touched or moved.

- The victim has difficulty moving the injured part.
- The injured part moves abnormally or unnaturally.
- The victim feels a grating sensation of bone ends rubbing together.
- The area of the injury is swollen.
- The injured part is deformed.
- The shape or length of a bone is different from the same bone on the other side of the body.
- The site of the injury shows a bluish discoloration.

WARNING

CHILD ABUSE

If you think a child is the victim of abuse, call a local child protective service agency, welfare department, public health department, or the police. (See p. 61.) You should suspect abuse if a child has any of the following:

- Fractures in the breastbone, back, skull, end of the collarbone, or the ribs in the back
- Multiple fractures in different stages of healing
- Fractures caused by twisting
- Recurring fractures in the same part of the body

WHAT TO DO

If the victim has a closed break:
1. Follow the steps on pp. 109–118 for immobilizing broken bones in specific parts of the body.
2. If the fracture is severe, call 911 (or your local emergency number). Otherwise, transport the victim yourself to the nearest hospital emergency department or doctor's office.

If the victim has an open break:
1. Call 911 (or your local emergency number) promptly.
2. Cut clothing away from the wound. *Do not* try to push back any part of the bone that is sticking out. *Do not* wash the wound or insert anything, including medication, into it.

3. *Gently* apply pressure with a large sterile or clean pad or cloth to stop the bleeding.
4. Cover the entire wound, including the protruding bone, with a bandage.
5. Apply splints if paramedics or other trained personnel are not readily available. Always splint the injured part by securing the splint above and below the injury before moving the victim. (See Splinting and Other Procedures, below.)
6. Handle the victim very gently. Rough handling often increases the severity of the injury.
7. *Do not* give the victim anything to eat or drink.

SPLINTING AND OTHER PROCEDURES

Splints are used to keep an injured part from moving, thereby easing pain and preventing the break from becoming worse. Objects that can be used for splinting include boards, straight sticks, brooms, pieces of corrugated cardboard bent to form a three-sided box, rolled newspapers or magazines, pillows, rolled blankets, skis or ski poles, oars, or umbrellas. Life jackets can be wrapped around knee or ankle injuries. If possible, the splint should extend beyond both the joint above and the joint below the broken bone. Padding, such as cloth, towels, or blankets, should be placed between the splint and the skin of the injured part.

Splints can be tied in place with neckties, strips of cloth torn from shirts, handkerchiefs, belts, string, rope, or other suitable material. *Do not* tie the splint so tightly that the ties interfere with circulation. Swelling or bluish discoloration of the fingers or toes may indicate that the ties are too tight and need to be loosened. Loosen splint ties if the victim experiences numbness or tingling or if he or she cannot move the fingers or toes. Check for a pulse and loosen the ties if no pulse can be felt.

Following are instructions on how to splint and treat breaks of specific bones. Keep in mind, however, that any suspected fracture needs to be evaluated by a doctor. After immobilizing a broken bone, take the person immediately to a hospital emergency department or doctor's office.

INJURIES AND ILLNESSES

Ankle Injury

WHAT TO DO

If the person cannot walk or move the ankle, if his or her toes are numb, or if the skin under the toenails is blue, take him or her immediately to the nearest hospital emergency department.

If the person does not have any of the above symptoms, follow the steps below for immobilizing the ankle before transporting him or her to a hospital emergency department or doctor's office:

1. Keep the victim lying down.
2. Remove the victim's shoe.
3. Place ties or strips under the leg. Place a pillow (preferably) or rolled blanket around the leg from the calf to well beyond the heel so that the pillow edges meet on top of the leg.

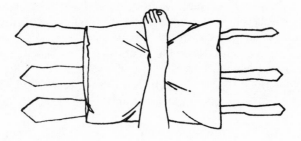

4. Fold the ends of the pillow that extend beyond the heel so that the pillow supports the foot and tie the pillow in place.

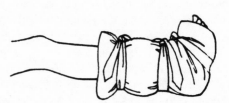

Upper Arm Injury

WHAT TO DO

If the person has no pulse in the wrist, cannot move his or her fingers or hand, cannot extend his or her hand at the wrist, or if his or her hand or fingers are numb, take him or her immediately to the nearest hospital emergency department.

If the person does not have any of the above symptoms, follow the steps below for immobilizing the arm before transporting him or her to a hospital emergency department or doctor's office:

1. Place some light padding in the victim's armpit and gently place the arm at the victim's side, with the lower part of the arm at a right angle across the victim's chest.

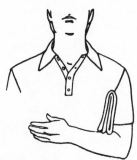

2. Make a padded splint out of newspaper or other material and apply it to the outside of the upper arm. Tie it in place above and below the break. Support the lower arm with a narrow sling tied around the neck.

3. Bind the upper arm to the victim's body by placing a large towel, bedsheet, or cloth around the splint and the victim's chest and tying it under the opposite arm.

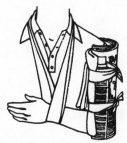

4. Have the victim sit up while riding to the hospital.

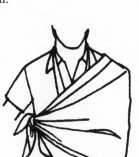

Lower Arm or Wrist Injury

WHAT TO DO

If the person has no pulse in the wrist or cannot move the fingers or if his or her fingers are numb or the skin under the fingernails is blue, take him or her immediately to the nearest hospital emergency department.

INJURIES AND ILLNESSES

If the person does not have any of the above symptoms, follow the steps below for immobilizing the arm before transporting him or her to a hospital emergency department or doctor's office:

1. Carefully place the lower arm at a right angle across the victim's chest with the palm facing toward the chest and the thumb pointing upward.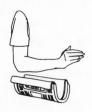
2. Apply a padded splint on each side of the lower arm, or use folded, padded newspapers or magazines wrapped under and around both sides of the arm. The splint should reach from the elbow to well beyond the wrist. Tie the splint in place above and below the break.
3. Support the lower arm with a wide sling tied around the neck. The sling should be placed so that the fingers are slightly higher (3 to 4 inches) than the level of the elbow.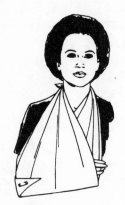
4. Have the victim sit up while riding to the hospital.

Collarbone Injury

WHAT TO DO

If the person has difficulty breathing or pain when breathing, an open wound in the chest, or numbness in the adjacent arm, call 911 (or your local emergency number) or take him or her immediately to the nearest hospital emergency department.

If the person does not have any of the above symptoms, follow the steps described in the illustration on p. 113 for immobilizing the collarbone before transporting him or her to a hospital emergency department or doctor's office:

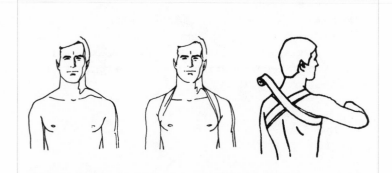

IMMOBILIZING THE COLLARBONE

Wrap an elastic bandage or other cloth (starting at the side of the neck) diagonally across the back, over the shoulder, under the arm and again diagonally across the back, over the shoulder, and under the arm. Repeat a few times. You should be able to slide one finger snugly under the ties in front. Illustration shows front and back views.

Elbow Injury

Elbow fractures often cause circulatory problems. Seek medical help at once if an elbow injury is suspected.

WHAT TO DO

If the person has no pulse in the wrist, cannot move his or her fingers or hand, or has numbness in the hand or fingers, take him or her immediately to the nearest hospital emergency department.

If the person does not have any of the above symptoms, follow the steps below for immobilizing the elbow before transporting him or her to a hospital emergency department or doctor's office:

If the elbow is bent:
1. *Do not* try to straighten the elbow.
2. Place the forearm in a sling and tie the sling around the victim's neck if possible.
3. If possible, bind the injured upper arm to the victim's body by placing a towel or cloth around the upper arm, sling, and chest and tying it under the victim's opposite arm.

INJURIES AND ILLNESSES

113

If the elbow is straight:
1. *Do not* try to bend the elbow to apply a sling.
2. Place padding in the victim's armpit.
3. Apply padded splints along one or both sides of the entire arm. If splints are not available, a pillow centered at the elbow and tied may be used.

Foot Injury

See: Ankle, p. 273.

Hand Injury

WHAT TO DO

If the person cannot move his or her fingers, if the skin under the fingernails is blue, or if the fingers are numb, take him or her immediately to the nearest hospital emergency department.

If the person does not have any of the above symptoms, follow the steps below for immobilizing the hand before transporting him or her to a hospital emergency department or doctor's office:

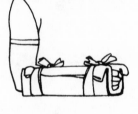

1. Bend the arm at the elbow
2. Place a padded splint underneath the lower arm and hand and tie the splint in place.
3. Place the lower arm against the victim's chest and put the lower arm into a sling and tie around the victim's neck.

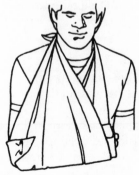

Kneecap Injury

WHAT TO DO

If the person's leg is numb below the level of the injury, if he or she is unable to walk or extend the leg, if the skin under the toenails is blue, or if the person has an open wound, take him or her immediately to the nearest hospital emergency department.

If the person does not have any of the above symptoms, follow the steps below for immobilizing the leg before transporting him or her to a hospital emergency department or doctor's office:

1. Gently straighten the victim's injured leg, if necessary.
2. Place a padded board at least 4 inches wide underneath the injured leg. The board should be long enough to reach from the victim's heel to the buttocks. Place extra padding under the ankle and knee.
3. Tie the splint in place at the ankle, just below and above the knee, and at the thigh. *Do not* tie over the kneecap.

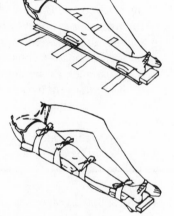

See Also: Dislocations, p. 151.

Thigh Injury

An injury to the thigh can cause internal bleeding, which can be life-threatening. If a person has had a severe blow to the thigh, or if you notice swelling or redness in the thigh, call 911 (or your local emergency number) or transport the person immediately to the nearest hospital emergency department.

WHAT TO DO

If the person's leg is numb below the level of the injury, if he or she is unable to walk or extend the leg, if the skin under the toenails is blue, or if the person has an open wound, take him or her immediately to the nearest hospital emergency department.

If the person does not have any of the above symptoms, follow the steps below for immobilizing the leg before transporting him or her to a hospital emergency department or doctor's office:

If board splints are not available:
1. Using traction (pull), carefully and slowly straighten the knee of the injured leg, if necessary.
2. Place padding, such as a folded blanket, between the victim's legs.
3. Tie the injured leg to the uninjured leg. Legs should be tied together in several places, including around the ankles, above and below the knees, and around the thighs. *Do not* tie directly over the break.

If board splints are available:
1. Using traction (pull), carefully and slowly straighten the knee of the injured leg if necessary.
2. Assemble about seven long bandages or cloth strips. Use a stick or small board to push each strip under the victim's body at a hollow such as the ankle, knee, or small of the back and then slide each strip into place (at the ankle; above and below the knee; at the thigh, pelvis, and lower back; and just below the armpit).
3. Place two well-padded splints in parallel position. The outside splint should be long enough to reach from the victim's armpit to below the heel. The inside splint should reach from the crotch to below the heel.
4. Tie the splints in place with knots at the outside splint.

Lower Leg Injury

WHAT TO DO

If the person's leg is numb below the level of the injury, if he or she is unable to walk or extend the leg, if the skin under the toenails is blue, or if the person has an open wound, take him or her immediately to the nearest hospital emergency department.

If the person does not have any of the above symptoms, follow these steps for immobilizing the leg before transporting him or her to a hospital emergency department or doctor's office:

If splints are not available:

1. Carefully and slowly straighten the injured leg, if necessary.
2. Place padding, such as a folded blanket, between the victim's legs.
3. Tie the legs together. (See Thigh Injury, p. 115.)

If splints are available:

1. Place a well-padded splint on each side of the injured leg. A third splint can be used underneath the leg. Splints should reach from above the knee to below the heel.
2. Tie the splints together in three or four places. *Do not* tie directly over the break.

To make a pillow splint:

1. Gently lift the injured leg and slide the pillow under the leg.
2. Bring the edges of the pillow to the top side of the leg. Pin the pillow together or tie the pillow around the leg in several places. For added support, place a rigid object such as a board or stick on each side of the pillow and fasten in place with ties above and below the suspected fracture site.

Neck Injury

See: Head, Neck, and Back Injuries (Neck Injuries), p. 197.

Pelvis Injury

WHAT TO DO

1. Call 911 (or your local emergency number) or transport the person immediately to the nearest hospital emergency department. An injury to the pelvis can cause severe internal bleeding and always requires evaluation by a doctor.
2. Keep the victim lying down on his or her back.
3. Legs may be straight or bent at the knees, whichever is more comfortable for the victim.
4. Tie the victim's legs together at the ankles and knees whether the legs are straight or bent.
5. If the victim must be taken to the hospital by someone other than trained medical personnel, place the victim on a well-

INJURIES AND ILLNESSES

padded rigid support such as a board, door, or table leaf. (See Head, Neck, and Back Injuries [Back Injuries], p. 201.)

Shoulder Injury

WHAT TO DO

If the person does not have a pulse in the wrist or if the shoulder injury was caused by a severe blow, take him or her immediately to the nearest hospital emergency department.

If the person does not have any of the above symptoms, follow the steps below for immobilizing the shoulder before transporting him or her to a hospital emergency department or doctor's office:

1. Place the victim's injured forearm at a right angle to his or her chest.
2. Apply a sling and tie around the victim's neck.
3. Bind the arm to the victim's body by placing a towel or cloth around the upper arm and chest and tying it under the victim's opposite arm.
4. Transport the victim to the nearest hospital emergency department. Have the victim sit up while riding to the hospital.

BRUISES

A bruise is the most common type of injury. It occurs when a fall or blow to the body causes small blood vessels to break beneath the skin. The discoloration and swelling in the skin are caused by the blood seeping into the tissues, which change colors as the bruise heals.

SYMPTOMS

Bruises can involve any or all of the following symptoms:

- Pain
- Area initially turns reddish-blue
- Area later turns green
- Lump (hematoma) may form
- Area becomes yellow then brown before fading

WARNING

CHILD ABUSE

If you think a child is the victim of abuse, call a local child protective service agency, welfare department, public health department, or the police. (See p. 61.) You should suspect abuse if a child has any of the following:

- Bruises in fleshy areas such as the face, back, abdomen, thighs, or buttocks
- Bruises in generally protected areas such as the neck, chest, or genitals
- Bruises with distinctive, recognizable shapes of objects such as cords, clothes hangers, or belt buckles
- Multiple bruises in various stages of healing
- Bruises around the neck (from choking)

INJURIES AND ILLNESSES

WHAT TO DO

1. As soon as possible, apply cold compresses or an ice bag to the affected area. Cold or ice decreases local bleeding and swelling.
2. If a bruise is on an arm or leg, elevate the limb above the level of the heart to decrease local blood flow.
3. After 24 hours, apply moist heat (a warm, wet compress) to aid healing. Heat dilates or opens blood vessels, increasing circulation to the affected area.
4. If the bruise is severe, or painful swelling develops, seek medical attention, as there is the possibility of a broken bone or other injury.

See Also: Bleeding, p. 96; Broken Bones, p. 107; Dislocations, p. 151; Lumps and Bumps, p. 216; Muscle Aches and Pains, p. 220; Sprains, p. 248.

The objectives of first aid for burns are to relieve pain, prevent infection, and prevent or treat for shock. Initial treatment of burns by the first-aider helps to decrease the temperature of the burned area. This, in turn, helps prevent further heat injury to the skin and underlying tissues.

Burns caused by fire, sunlight, or hot substances are classified according to the degree of the injury. First-degree burns are the least dangerous. Third-degree burns are the most serious.

WARNING

CHILD ABUSE

If you think a child is the victim of abuse, call a local child protective service agency, welfare department, public health department, or the police. (See p. 61.) You should suspect abuse if a child has any of the following:

- A burn with a distinctive, recognizable pattern of an object such as a grid, hot plate, or light bulb
- Multiple circular burns from cigarettes
- A burn with the pattern of a glove or stocking on an arm or leg, or a clear-cut, sharp edge from being immersed in scalding water
- Multiple burns in various stages of healing

FIRST-DEGREE BURNS

A burn resulting in injury only to the outside layer of the skin is a first-degree burn. Sunburn and brief contact with hot objects, hot water, or steam are common causes of first-degree burns and cause no blistering of the burned areas. First-degree burns usually heal within a week.

SYMPTOMS

First-degree burns can cause any or all of the following symptoms:

- Redness
- Mild swelling
- Pain
- Unbroken skin (no blisters)

WHAT TO DO

1. Immediately put the burned area under cool running water or apply a cool-water compress (a clean towel, washcloth, or handkerchief soaked in cool water) until pain decreases.
2. Cover the burn with nonfluffy sterile or clean bandages. *Do not* apply butter or grease to a burn. Do not apply medications or home remedies without a doctor's recommendation.

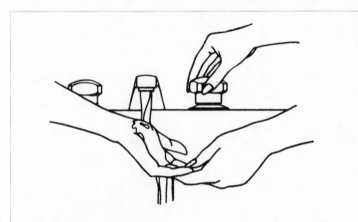

TREATING A BURN
To lower the temperature of the burned area and stop further skin damage, immediately put the burned area under cool running water or apply cool-water compresses until pain subsides.

SECOND-DEGREE BURNS

A burn that causes injury to the layers of skin beneath the surface of the body is a second-degree burn. Deep sunburn, hot liquids, and flash burns from gasoline and other substances are common causes of second-degree burns. Healing may take up to 3 weeks.

SYMPTOMS

Second-degree burns can cause any or all of the following symptoms:

- Redness, or a blotchy or streaky appearance
- Blisters
- Swelling that lasts for several days
- Moist, oozy appearance of the surface of the skin
- Pain

WHAT TO DO

1. Put the burned area in cool (not iced) water or apply cool-water compresses (a clean towel, washcloth, or handkerchief soaked in cool water) until pain subsides. Any cool liquid you can drink—such as water, a soft drink, beer, or a milk shake—can be poured on a burn. Even room-temperature tap water will work. The purpose is to decrease the temperature of the burned skin as quickly as possible and limit tissue damage. Do not apply ice.
2. Gently pat the area dry with a clean towel or other soft material.
3. Remove any constricting jewelry.
4. Cover the burned area with a dry, nonfluffy sterile bandage or clean cloth to prevent infection. *Do not* attempt to break blisters or apply ointments, sprays, antiseptics, or home remedies.
5. Elevate burned arms or legs.
6. Seek medical attention. If the victim has flash burns around the lips or nose, or has singed nasal hairs, breathing problems may develop. Seek medical attention immediately, preferably at the nearest hospital emergency department.

INJURIES AND ILLNESSES

WARNING

Victims who have inhaled smoke or other substances can develop lung damage and should seek immediate medical attention. Prompt medical attention is also required for burns that cover more than 15 percent of the body of an adult or 10 percent of the body of a child, or for burns on the face, hands, or feet. To determine the percentage of the burned area, an easy rule is that the victim's palm represents 1 percent of his or her body area.

THIRD-DEGREE BURNS

A burn that destroys all layers of the skin is a third-degree burn. Fire, prolonged contact with hot substances, and electrical burns are common causes of third-degree burns.

SYMPTOMS

Third-degree burns may cause any or all of the following symptoms:

- White or leathery skin at burn site
- Skin damage
- Little pain (because nerve endings have been destroyed)

WARNING

- *Do not* remove clothes that are stuck to the burn.
- *Do not* put ice or ice water on burns. This can intensify the shock reaction.
- *Do not* apply ointments, sprays, antiseptics, or home remedies to burns.

WHAT TO DO

1. If the victim is on fire, smother the flames with a blanket, bedspread, rug, or jacket.

2. Call 911 (or your local emergency number) or take the victim to the nearest hospital emergency department. It is very important that victims with even *small* third-degree burns consult a doctor.

3. Check often to see if the victim has trouble breathing and maintain an open airway if breathing becomes difficult. Breathing difficulties are common with burns, particularly with burns around the face, neck, and mouth, and with smoke inhalation.

4. Place a cool cloth or cool (not iced) water on burns of the face, hands, or feet to cool the burned areas.

5. Cover the burned area with thick, sterile, nonfluffy dressings. A clean sheet, pillowcase, or disposable diaper can be used.

6. Elevate burned hands higher than the victim's heart, if possible.

7. Elevate burned legs or feet. Do not allow the victim to walk.

8. If the victim has face or neck burns, he or she should be propped up with pillows.

9. Watch for signs of shock, such as a fast and weak pulse and fast breathing. If the victim is in shock, do the following while waiting for medical help to arrive:

- Keep the victim lying down unless the face or neck is burned.
- Elevate the victim's feet 8 to 12 inches unless the victim is unconscious or has neck, spine, head, chest, or severe lower face or jaw injuries. A victim who is unconscious or who has severe lower face or jaw injuries should be placed on his or her side (not facedown) with the head slightly extended to prevent choking on fluids or vomit. If the victim is having trouble breathing, elevate his or her head and shoulders slightly.
- If pain increases, lower the feet again.
- Keep the victim comfortably warm but not hot, covered with a blanket or coat. If possible, place a blanket beneath a victim who is on the ground.
- *Do not* give fluids by mouth.
- Calm and reassure the victim. Gentleness, kindness, and understanding play an important role in treating a victim in shock.

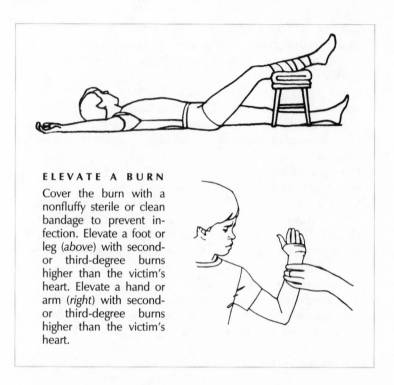

ELEVATE A BURN
Cover the burn with a nonfluffy sterile or clean bandage to prevent infection. Elevate a foot or leg (*above*) with second- or third-degree burns higher than the victim's heart. Elevate a hand or arm (*right*) with second- or third-degree burns higher than the victim's heart.

CHEMICAL BURNS

WHAT TO DO

1. Quickly flush the burned area with large quantities of running water for 5 to 10 minutes. Speed and quantity of water are both important in minimizing the extent of the injury. Use a garden hose, buckets of water, a shower, or a tub. Do not use a strong stream of water if it can be avoided.
2. Continue to flush with water while removing clothing from the burned area.
3. After flushing, follow the instructions on the label of the chemical that caused the burn, if available.
4. Cover the burn with a nonfluffy clean bandage or clean cloth. *Do not* apply ointments, sprays, antiseptics, or home remedies. Cool wet dressings are best for pain.
5. Seek immediate medical attention.

TAR AND ASPHALT BURNS

The large pots in which workers mix tar and asphalt at the back of roofing trucks maintain temperatures of up to 500°F. Spills or contact with tar or asphalt directly from the pot can cause severe, third-degree burns. When spread on a roof, the material is somewhat cooler but is still hot enough to cause second-degree burns.

WHAT TO DO

1. Apply cold water to the burned area to harden the tar.
2. Spread petroleum jelly on gauze or a soft cloth and wipe it over the area to remove the tar. Do not use gasoline, acetone, or kerosene to clean the burn.
3. Seek immediate medical attention.

See Also: Electrical Burns, p. 168; Heat-Related Problems, p. 206; Seizures, p. 237; Shock, p. 240.

INJURIES AND ILLNESSES

CARBON MONOXIDE
POISONING

Carbon monoxide—a colorless, odorless, tasteless gas—is a common cause of poisoning death. Most accidental cases of carbon monoxide poisoning occur in the home during the winter months, usually at night when people are sleeping. The gas can be produced by any source of heat or fire that is enclosed without proper ventilation and is present in the exhaust of motor vehicles. Sources of carbon monoxide in the home include faulty forced-air gas furnaces or other gas appliances, unventilated space heaters, poorly ventilated fireplaces, and indoor cooking with grills that use charcoal or chemical fuels.

Be extremely cautious when rescuing a victim from an area filled with smoke or chemical or gas fumes. Do not attempt a rescue alone. Before entering the area, rapidly inhale and exhale two or three times; take a deep breath and hold it. Remain close to the ground (crawl) while entering and rescuing the victim so that you will not inhale hot air or fumes. If the area is extremely hot or heavy with fumes, it is best to leave the rescue to someone who has an independent air supply. Do nothing at the site but remove the victim.

SYMPTOMS

Poisoning from carbon monoxide or other dangerous fumes can cause any or all of the following symptoms, which are sometimes confused with the symptoms of food poisoning (in an infant, the only noticeable symptoms are often irritability and lethargy):

- Headache
- Dizziness
- Nausea
- Weakness and light-headedness
- Inability to move or concentrate
- Chest pain

- Shortness of breath
- Seizures
- Coma

WHAT TO DO

1. Get the victim into fresh air immediately (upwind of the poisonous fumes).
2. Maintain an open airway. Restore breathing and circulation if necessary. (See pp. 31–50.)
3. Loosen tight clothing around the victim's neck and waist.
4. Seek medical attention immediately even if the victim seems to partially or completely recover. Call 911 (or your local emergency number) and inform medics of the need for oxygen.

Preventing Carbon Monoxide Poisoning

Here are some steps you can take to help keep your family safe from carbon monoxide poisoning:

- Install carbon monoxide detectors (available at hardware and houseware stores) on each floor of your home, including every bedroom. (Most cases of carbon monoxide poisoning occur at night while sleeping.)
- Make sure that all furnaces and gas appliances are properly installed and adequately ventilated.
- Have all furnaces and gas appliances inspected and maintained every year by a trained professional.
- Do not burn fuels such as gas or kerosene in confined spaces or rooms. Never use a barbecue grill indoors.
- Make sure that space heaters are adequately ventilated.

INJURIES AND ILLNESSES

CHILDBIRTH, EMERGENCY

Occasionally, childbirth occurs at an unexpected time or labor proceeds more quickly than expected. In such cases, the mother sometimes cannot get to the hospital in time for the delivery. If the mother's contractions are 2 to 3 minutes apart, if she feels the urge to push down, or if the baby's head is visible in the vaginal opening (about the size of a half-dollar or larger), birth will usually occur very soon.

If at all possible, summon a doctor to deliver the infant. Sometimes a doctor can give instructions over the telephone during the delivery. Try to remain calm. Most births occur naturally and normally. *Do not* try to delay or prevent the birth of the baby by crossing the mother's legs or pushing on the baby's head or by any other means. This could be very harmful to the infant.

PREPARATION AND DELIVERY

Before the Baby Arrives

WHAT TO DO

1. Place clean sheets on the bed. If time allows, a shower curtain or rubber sheet placed underneath the clean linen will help protect the mattress. If a bed is not available, place clean cloths, clothes, or newspapers underneath the mother's hips and thighs on the floor or ground. A fresh newspaper is generally very clean and almost sterile.
2. Have the mother lie on her back with her knees bent, her feet flat, and her knees and thighs wide apart.
3. Sterilize scissors or a knife in boiling water for at least 5 minutes if possible or hold over a flame for 30 seconds. Leave the scissors or knife in the water until you are ready to use it. Either may be used to cut the umbilical cord.

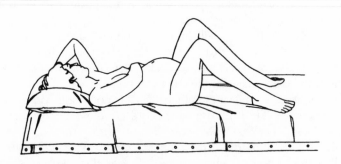

PREPARING FOR DELIVERY

Place clean sheets on the bed. If no bed is available, place clean cloths, clothes, or newspapers underneath the mother's hips and thighs on the floor, leaving room for the birth of the baby. Have the mother lie on her back with her knees bent, her feet flat, and her knees and thighs wide apart.

4. Gather together:

- Clean, soft, cotton blanket, sheet, or towel to wrap the baby
- Clean, strong string or clean shoelaces, cord, or strips of cloth to tie off the umbilical cord
- Pail or bucket in case the mother vomits
- Large plastic bag, container, or towel in which to place the afterbirth (placenta) for later inspection by medical personnel
- Sanitary napkins or clean, folded cloths or handkerchiefs to be placed over the vagina after the birth of the baby and after the delivery of the afterbirth
- Diapers and safety pins

Delivering the Baby

WHAT TO DO

1. Wash your hands with soap and water. *Do not* place your hands or other objects in the vagina. *Do not* interfere with the delivery or touch the baby until the head is completely out of the vagina. Usually the baby will be born facedown.

131

2. Once the baby's head is out, guide and support it to keep it free of blood and other secretions.

3. If the baby's head is still inside a liquid-filled bag, carefully puncture the bag with the sterile scissors or your finger and open it to allow the fluid to escape. Remove the membranes from the baby's face so the baby can breathe.

4. Check to make sure the umbilical cord is not wrapped around the baby's neck. If the umbilical cord is *not* wrapped around the baby's neck, do not worry about cutting the cord until after the baby's birth. If the umbilical cord is wrapped around the baby's neck, gently and quickly slip the cord over the baby's head. If the cord is wrapped too tightly to slip over the baby's head, the cord must be cut *now* to prevent the baby from strangling. If you have cut the cord and if someone is available to help you, have that individual tie off the umbilical cord ends. (See Immediate Care of the Baby, number 8, p. 134.)

5. Continue to support the head as the baby is being born. The baby will be very slippery, so be gentle and very careful.

6. Once the baby's head and neck are out of the vagina, the baby will turn on his or her side to allow passage of the shoulders. The upper shoulder usually emerges first. Carefully and gently guide the baby's head slightly downward. Once the upper shoulder is out, gently lift the baby's head upward to allow the lower shoulder to emerge. *Do not* pull the child out by the armpits.

7. Carefully hold the slippery baby as the rest of his or her body slides out.

Immediate Care of the Baby

WHAT TO DO

1. To help the baby start breathing, hold the baby with his or her head lower than the feet so that secretions can drain from the lungs, mouth, and nose. Support the head and body with one hand while grasping the baby's legs at the ankles with the other hand.

2. Wipe out the mouth and nose gently with sterile gauze or a clean cloth to make sure that nothing interferes with breathing.

3. If the baby has not yet cried, slap your fingers against the bottom of the baby's feet or gently rub the baby's back.
4. If the baby is still not breathing, give artificial respiration through *both* the baby's mouth and nose, keeping the head extended. (See pp. 32–33.) Give very gentle puffs every 3 seconds.

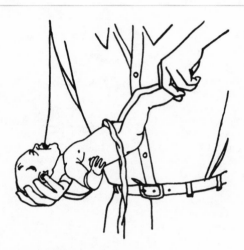

AFTER THE DELIVERY
After the baby is born, hold the baby with his or her head lower than the feet so that secretions can drain from the lungs, mouth, and nose. Support the head and body with one hand while grasping the baby's legs and ankles with the other hand.

5. Note the time of delivery.
6. Once the baby starts breathing, wrap him or her, including the top and back of his or her head, in a blanket or sheet to prevent heat loss. Place the baby on his or her side on the mother's stomach with the baby's head slightly lower than the rest of the body and facing the mother's feet. The umbilical cord should be kept loose. It is very important to keep the baby warm and breathing well.

   Do not clean the white cheesy coating covering the baby's skin. This is a protective covering. *Do not* clean the baby's eyes or ears.
7. It is not necessary or desirable to cut the umbilical cord immediately. It is best to wait about a minute, until the cord

stops pulsating. If the mother can be taken to the hospital immediately after the delivery of the afterbirth (which occurs 5 to 20 minutes after delivery of the baby), the baby can be left attached to the umbilical cord and afterbirth, particularly if there are no clean scissors to cut the cord. Also, the cord must be cut properly.

TYING THE UMBILICAL CORD

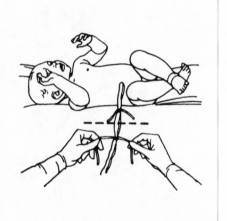

If the umbilical cord is to be cut, tie a clean string around the cord at least 4 inches from the baby's body. Tie in a tight square knot so that circulation is cut off in the cord. Use a second piece of string to tie another tight square knot 6 to 8 inches from the baby (2 to 4 inches from the first knot). Cut the cord between the two ties.

8. If you must cut the cord, tie a clean string or strip of cloth around the cord at least 4 inches from the baby's body. Tie the string in a tight square knot so that circulation is cut off in the cord. Using a second piece of string or strip of cloth, tie another tight square knot 6 to 8 inches from the baby (2 to 4 inches from the first knot).

9. Cut the cord between the two ties with sterilized or clean scissors or a knife.

10. Keep the baby warm with his or her head covered and close to the mother. The baby's head should still be slightly lower than the rest of his or her body to allow drainage of secretions.

DELIVERY OF THE AFTERBIRTH

Delivery of the afterbirth (placenta) usually occurs 5 to 20 minutes after the birth of the baby. It is usually preceded by a gush of dark red blood from the vagina.

1. Be patient in waiting for the delivery of the afterbirth. *Do not* pull on the umbilical cord to quicken delivery of the afterbirth. The mother's uterine contractions will eventually push out the afterbirth.
2. Place the afterbirth in a container and take it with the mother and baby to the hospital so that it may be examined.

CARE OF THE MOTHER

After the infant has been born and the afterbirth has been expelled:

1. Place sanitary napkins or clean, folded cloths against the mother's vaginal opening to absorb blood.
2. To help control the flow of blood from the mother, place your hands on the mother's abdomen and gently massage the uterus, which can be felt just below the mother's navel and feels like a large smooth ball. Continue to massage gently until the uterus feels firm. Continue to do this every 5 minutes or so for an hour, unless medical assistance is obtained. If the bleeding is very heavy and/or prolonged, seek medical attention immediately.
3. If she wishes, sponge the mother's face with cool water.
4. Give the mother water, tea, coffee, or broth. *Do not* give her alcoholic beverages.
5. Keep the mother warm and comfortable. And remember, congratulations are in order!

MEDICAL ATTENTION

Regardless of how smoothly the delivery goes, it is very important that both the mother and baby be examined by a physician to make certain all is well. Most serious problems occur in the first 24 hours after birth.

See Also: Miscarriage, p. 219; Pregnancy Danger Signs, p. 228.

INJURIES AND ILLNESSES

CHILLS

Chills may be a symptom of many medical problems, including flu, kidney and bladder infections, bacterial pneumonia, food poisoning, and spider bites. Chills are also associated with exposure to cold.

Chills are nature's way of raising the body temperature. Chills occur when there is decreased blood circulation to the body surface due to narrowing of the blood vessels in the skin. Muscles in the body contract. Shivering and shaking associated with chills produce heat in the body, thus allowing the body temperature to rise. Often, chills are followed by fever and indicate the onset of an infection.

> **WARNING**
>
> CHILLS BROUGHT ON BY MEDICATION
>
> Call 911 (or your local emergency number) or take the person to the nearest emergency department if the chills and tremors are associated with taking tranquilizers or antidepressants. This situation can indicate a life-threatening imbalance of chemicals in the brain and nervous system.

WHAT TO DO

1. Make the victim comfortably warm but do not use hot water bottles or heating pads.
2. Offer warm drinks and liquids such as tea or soup if the victim is not nauseated or vomiting.
3. Seek medical attention; a serious infection may be present.

See Also: Bites and Stings (Spider and Tick Bites), p. 76; Cold-Related Problems, p. 139; Fever, p. 180; Food Poisoning, p. 185; Heat-Related Problems, p. 206.

The Heimlich maneuver (abdominal thrust) is the method of choice to use in an emergency situation when a person is choking. Back blows—hitting the victim forcefully and repeatedly between the shoulder blades with the palm of your hand—are used on adults and children only if the Heimlich maneuver has not been effective in dislodging a foreign object from the windpipe (trachea).

SYMPTOMS

Perform the Heimlich maneuver following steps on pp. 51–56 if you are with someone who has any or all of the following symptoms:

- Gasping or breathing noisily and/or coughing
- Grasping his or her throat
- Unable to talk
- Pale, white, gray, or blue skin
- Unconsciousness
- Breathing stops

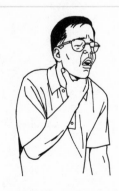

CHOKING SIGN
A person who is choking will involuntarily grasp his or her neck.

INJURIES AND ILLNESSES

CHOKING IN CHILDREN

Occasionally, children will swallow pieces of food or small objects—usually nuts, hot dogs, hard candy, raisins, grapes, coins, small toys, or batteries—that lodge in the upper airway above or between the vocal cords. The lodged object may cause the child's voice to sound strained or strangely mechanical.

WHAT TO DO

1. If a piece of food or other object becomes lodged in the child's throat and the child is able to cough or is breathing noisily, he or she will make involuntary attempts to cough out the object. *Do not* interfere with the child's efforts to cough out the object and *do not* stick your fingers down the child's throat, as this may cause the object to become lodged even farther.
2. Watch the child carefully and remain as calm as possible so that you do not frighten him or her.
3. If the child is unable to cough out the lodged particle, take him or her to a doctor's office or hospital emergency department. Stay with the child at all times, remain calm, and provide reassurance.
4. Perform the Heimlich maneuver immediately following the steps on pp. 52–53 for a child over 1 or the steps on p. 54 for an infant under 1 if symptoms continue and one or more of the following happens:

   - Grasping at the throat (an involuntary movement that indicates choking)
   - Extreme difficulty breathing
   - Skin and lips turn blue

See Also: Unconsciousness, p. 259.

COLD-RELATED PROBLEMS

FROSTBITE

Frostbite is freezing of parts of the body due to exposure to very low temperatures. Frostbite occurs when ice crystals form in the fluid in the cells of the skin and other tissues. The toes, fingers, nose, and ears are affected most often. A person is more susceptible to frostbite if he or she is in cold, windy weather after consuming alcohol or getting his or her skin wet.

SYMPTOMS

Frostbite can cause any or all of the following symptoms:

- Redness and stinging, burning pain (in early stages)
- White or grayish yellow, waxy-looking skin (in later stages); swelling; throbbing
- Coldness and numbness
- Absence of pain (in later stages)
- Blisters

WARNING

SEVERE FROSTBITE

If severe frostbite has occurred, the victim may not have feeling in the frostbitten areas and they may be black, which indicates that the skin tissue has died. In this case, cover the frostbitten areas with warm materials and take the victim *without delay* to the nearest hospital emergency department for treatment.

WHAT TO DO

1. While outside, cover the frozen part with extra clothing or a warm cloth. If the hand or fingers are frostbitten, put the hand under the armpit for additional warmth. *Do not* rub the frostbitten part with snow or anything else.
2. Bring the victim inside promptly and remove any wet, cold, or constricting clothing from the frostbitten area.
3. Rewarm the frostbitten area rapidly (which will probably cause some pain). Put the victim's frostbitten part in warm (not hot) water that is between 104°F and 108°F. Test the water with a thermometer or by applying it to your forearm. Rewarming usually takes about half an hour.
4. If warm water is not available, gently wrap the frostbitten part in blankets or other warm, dry materials. *Do not* use heat lamps, hot water bottles, or heating pads. *Do not* allow the victim to place the frostbitten part near a hot stove or radiator (frostbitten parts could become burned because of the lack of pain sensation).
5. Put sterile gauze between frostbitten fingers or toes to keep them separated. Keep the frostbitten parts elevated, if possible.
6. Give the victim warm drinks such as tea, coffee, or soup. *Do not* give alcoholic beverages.
7. Stop the warming process when the skin becomes its normal color and/or feeling begins to come back. *Do not* break blisters. Ibuprofen may help relieve the pain.
8. Have the victim move the fingers or toes as soon as they are warmed. *Do not* allow a victim with frostbitten feet or toes to walk. This may cause further damage to the frostbitten part.
9. Seek medical attention promptly.
10. Take extreme care that the frostbitten area is not exposed to cold until it has thawed completely.

HYPOTHERMIA

Hypothermia is chilling of the entire body to 95°F. Hypothermia may result from immersion in very cold water, prolonged exposure to extremely cold weather, or wearing damp clothing in very cold conditions.

SYMPTOMS

Hypothermia can cause any or all of the following symptoms:

- Shivering
- Numbness
- Drowsiness or sleepiness
- Muscle weakness
- Dizziness
- Nausea

- Low body temperature
- Unconsciousness, if entire body is severely chilled or frozen
- Weak, slow pulse
- Large pupils

WHAT TO DO

1. Call 911 (or your local emergency number). Maintain an open airway. Restore breathing and circulation if necessary. (See pp. 31–50.)
2. Bring the victim into a warm room as soon as possible.
3. Remove wet clothes.
4. Have the victim lie down and wrap him or her in warm blankets, a sleeping bag, towels, additional clothing, or sheets. *Do not* massage the arms or legs because you could worsen any muscle damage.
5. If the victim is conscious, give him or her comfortably warm drinks such as hot chocolate, soup, or warm gelatin. *Do not* give the victim alcoholic beverages.
6. Check and treat for frostbite (p. 139) if necessary.

MILD CHILLING

For mild chilling, put the victim in a warm room and wrap him or her in warm blankets. Give the victim warm drinks such as coffee, tea, or soup. *Do not* give the victim alcoholic beverages.

Preventing Cold-Related Problems

Here are some steps you can take to avoid frostbite and other problems during cold weather:

- Wear polyester (not cotton) underwear and several layers of loose-fitting clothing. Goose down, polypropylene, wool, and polyester are all good insulating materials.

INJURIES AND ILLNESSES

141

- Do not wear tight, constricting socks or boots. Wear thin socks against your skin and one or two pairs of heavier outer socks.
- Try to keep your hands and feet dry and avoid sweating.
- Wear mittens instead of gloves; mittens should be loose.
- Never touch metal objects with your bare skin.
- Never travel or work alone out of doors in extremely cold weather.
- Avoid dehydration by drinking plenty of fluids.
- Avoid alcohol, barbiturates, and cigarettes.
- If you are an older person, set your indoor thermostat above 70°F. Consider using an electric blanket for sleeping.

See Also: Ear Problems (Frostbitten Ears), p. 166; Unconsciousness, p. 259.

DECOMPRESSION SICKNESS

Decompression sickness, also known as the bends, occurs when an individual rises too quickly from a compressed atmosphere (such as very deep water) to a higher altitude. Doing so can cause air bubbles—mostly nitrogen—to form in the blood. An air bubble that travels to the brain can cause instant death. The condition occurs in varying degrees of severity usually in inexperienced divers and, rarely, in miners.

SYMPTOMS

Decompression sickness may cause any or all of the following symptoms:

- Itchy rash, especially on the trunk, ears, wrists, or hands
- Blotchy purple rash near the waist
- Numbness and/or tingling, especially around the waist
- Dizziness or ringing in the ears
- Nausea or vomiting
- Pain that causes the person to bend over
- Difficulty breathing
- Paralysis
- Bleeding from the nose or ears
- Pain in the joints

WHAT TO DO

If the person is not breathing:
1. Call 911 (or your local emergency number) or take the person to the nearest hospital emergency department. The victim will need immediate medical attention (oxygen therapy).
2. Maintain an open airway. Restore breathing and circulation if necessary. (See pp. 31–50.)

If the person is breathing but unconscious:

1. Place him or her on his or her side to prevent choking on vomit.
2. Call 911 (or your local emergency number) or take the person to the nearest hospital emergency department. The victim will need immediate medical attention (oxygen therapy).

Preventing Decompression Sickness

If you have heart disease or a lung condition, do not dive without talking to your doctor first. Here are some steps you can take to avoid decompression sickness:

- Avoid dehydration by drinking plenty of fluids before diving.
- Do shallow dives.
- Ascend slowly (no faster than 16 to 23 feet per minute).
- If you have had an episode of decompression sickness, do not dive again for at least 4 weeks.

Dehydration is lack of adequate water in the body. Severe dehydration can occur with vomiting, excessive heat and sweating, diarrhea, or lack of food or fluid intake. Dehydration is a medical emergency and can be fatal. The condition is common in the elderly and can occur rapidly in infants and young children. Each year nearly 500 American children under 4 years old die of dehydration resulting from diarrhea.

SYMPTOMS

Dehydration may cause any or all of the following symptoms:

- Extreme thirst (that the victim may not be able to quench)
- Tiredness
- Light-headedness
- Abdominal or muscle cramping
- Restlessness

WHAT TO DO

1. Move the victim into the shade or a cool area.
2. Replace lost fluids and body chemicals by giving the victim water, carbonated beverages that have been allowed to go flat, a commercial electrolyte-replacement drink, flavored gelatin (in liquid form), or clear broth. Avoid low-sodium broth and caffeinated beverages.
3. Seek medical attention if symptoms persist or if complications arise (see warning box).

See Also: Diarrhea, p. 148; Heat-Related Problems, p. 206; Seizures, p. 237; Vomiting, p. 262.

INJURIES AND ILLNESSES

WARNING

SEVERE DEHYDRATION

Call 911 (or your local emergency number) or take the person to the nearest emergency department if you notice any or all of the following signs of severe dehydration:

- Vomiting or diarrhea
- Seizures
- Fast, weak pulse
- Fast breathing
- Sunken eyes
- Lack of tears
- Wrinkled fingers or toes
- Dry mouth

DIABETIC COMA

Diabetic coma is a life-threatening condition that can occur in people who have diabetes when the level of the sugar-regulating hormone insulin in their blood is too low. Insulin levels can go down to dangerous levels in people with diabetes if their body is not using the hormone properly—usually because they have missed an injection of insulin, they are not eating properly, or they have an infection.

SYMPTOMS

A diabetic coma can cause any or all of the following symptoms (which usually come on gradually):

- Extreme thirst
- Warm, red, dry skin
- Drowsiness
- Fruity-smelling breath
- Deep, rapid breathing
- Dry mouth and tongue
- Nausea with upper abdominal discomfort
- Vomiting
- Frequent urination
- Fast heart rate

WHAT TO DO

Call 911 (or your local emergency number) or take the person to the nearest hospital emergency department.

See Also: Unconsciousness, p. 259; Vomiting, p. 262.

Diarrhea—frequent loose, watery bowel movements—has many causes. The most common include food poisoning, certain medications, emotional stress, excessive drinking, and viral and bacterial infections.

If diarrhea is not severe and the individual can and will drink liquids, the body can replace lost fluids. If the individual can't or won't drink liquids or is vomiting, replacement of fluids will be impossible and dehydration can occur rapidly. Hospitalization may be necessary.

DIARRHEA IN ADULTS

SYMPTOMS

Diarrhea is characterized by any or all of the following symptoms:

- Frequent loose and watery stools (stools may vary from light tan to green)
- Stomach cramping
- Tiredness (due to loss of potassium)
- Thirst (due to loss of fluid)
- Blood streaks in or on stools

WHAT TO DO

1. A liquid diet is recommended to replace lost fluids and some body chemicals. Drink clear broth, a commercial electrolyte-replacement drink, flavored gelatin (in liquid form), carbonated beverages that have been allowed to go flat, or a sugar and salt solution (see p. 150). Water alone may pass right through the body. Drink at least 8 ounces of the solution every hour. Do not eat solid foods for about 24 hours.

2. If diarrhea persists longer than a day or two, or if urine decreases in both frequency and amount, seek medical attention immediately because fatal dehydration may occur.

WARNING

DEHYDRATION

For either an adult or a child with diarrhea, if symptoms continue or the following signs of severe dehydration appear, take the person immediately to the nearest hospital emergency department:

- Three or four loose, watery bowel movements every 4 to 6 hours
- Fever
- Dry mouth
- Decreased urination in both frequency and amount
- Drowsiness and sluggishness
- Sunken eyes
- Vomiting
- Black, tarry stool
- Blood or mucus in stool
- Weak cry (in children)
- Severe or prolonged stomach cramps

DIARRHEA IN CHILDREN

Common causes of diarrhea in infants and children are infection, spoiled food, food allergies or intolerance, foods with laxative effects, and poisoning.

If diarrhea is not severe and the child can and will drink liquids, the body can replace lost fluids. If the child can't or won't drink liquids or is vomiting, replacement of fluids will be impossible and dehydration can occur rapidly, especially in children under 5 years. Hospitalization may be necessary.

INJURIES AND ILLNESSES

SYMPTOMS

Frequent loose, watery bowel movements, which may or may not have a bad odor.

WHAT TO DO

1. Give the child liquids to replace lost fluids and some body chemicals. Do not give fruit juice or milk, however, because they can make the condition worse. Have the child drink clear broth, flavored gelatin (in liquid form), or carbonated beverages that have been allowed to go flat. Water alone may pass right through the body. Call the doctor before giving an electrolyte-replacement drink or a sugar and salt solution (see below) to ask how much to give.
2. Do not give the child solid foods for 24 hours.

Sugar and Salt Solution

1 quart of water
1 tablespoon of sugar
4 teaspoons of cream of tartar
1 teaspoon of salt
½ teaspoon of baking soda

Mix the ingredients. If cream of tartar and baking soda are not available, use just the water, sugar, and salt.

See Also: Dehydration, p. 145; Food Poisoning, p. 185; Vomiting, p. 262.

A dislocation occurs when the end of a bone is displaced from its joint. It usually results from a fall or a blow to the bone. Common areas of dislocations include the shoulder, hip, elbow, fingers, thumb, and kneecap. One of the most frequent dislocations is a pulled elbow in children under 5 years. The dislocation usually occurs when a child's arm is pulled up by the wrist, causing one of the forearm bones to slip out of place.

SYMPTOMS

Dislocations may cause any or all of the following symptoms:

- Swelling
- Deformity
- Pain on moving the injured part or inability to move the part
- Discoloration
- Tenderness
- Numbness

WHAT TO DO

1. *Do not* move or try to put a dislocated bone back into its place. Unskilled handling can cause extensive damage to nerves and blood vessels. The bone may be fractured and any movement may cause further tissue damage.
2. Place the victim in a comfortable position.
3. Immobilize the injured part with a splint, pillow, or sling in the position in which it was found. (See Broken Bones [Splinting and Other Procedures], p. 109.)
4. Seek medical attention promptly, preferably at the nearest hospital emergency department.

See Also: Broken Bones, p. 107; Sprains, p. 248; Wounds, p. 264; and Sports First Aid (pp. 271–336).

INJURIES AND ILLNESSES

DROWNING

In all emergencies involving a drowning person, remember first to be careful for your own safety. In deep water, a drowning person can drag a rescuer under water. Keep calm and do not overestimate your strength. If another person is with you, have that person call for help.

People who have been submerged in cold water (below 70°F) often can survive without brain damage. Some victims have been submerged for as long as 38 minutes and have lived. A reflex most prominent in young children slows the heartbeat and reserves the oxygen in the blood for the heart and brain. Mouth-to-mouth breathing and CPR must be started as soon as possible and continued, often for several hours, until the victim's body has become warm and he or she begins breathing on his or her own. Further medical treatment at a doctor's office or hospital emergency department will also be necessary.

HOW TO RESCUE FROM WATER

Do not move a victim with a suspected neck injury unless the victim's life and yours are in danger. Any movement of the head, either forward, backward, or side to side, can result in paralysis or death. If you must move the victim, always keep the head, neck, and body in alignment. (See p. 197.)

If a drowning victim is near a pier or the side of a swimming pool, lie down and give the victim your hand or foot and pull him or her to safety. If the victim is too far away, hold out a life preserver ring, pole, stick, board, rope, chair, tree limb, towel, or other object.

If the victim is out from the shore, wade into the water and extend a pole, board, stick, or rope to the victim and pull him or her to safety. It may be necessary to row a boat to the victim. If so, hand the victim an oar or other suitable object and pull him or

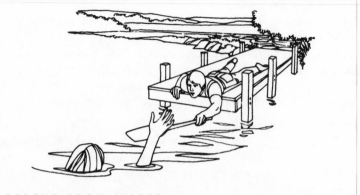

RESCUE FROM WATER

If a drowning victim is near a pier, but too far away to reach your hand or foot, lie down and hold out a pole, paddle, or life preserver, and pull the victim to safety.

her to the boat. If possible, the victim should hold on to the back of the boat while being rowed to the shore. If this is not possible, pull the victim carefully into the boat.

WHAT TO DO

If a neck or back injury is suspected (from a diving or surfboard accident):
If trained medical personnel are not available to assist you, place a board (such as a surfboard or table leaf) under the victim's head and back while he or she is still in the water. (The board should extend from the head to at least the buttocks.) This will keep the victim from moving, thus preventing further damage to the neck or back. Lift the victim out of the water on the board.

If the victim is not breathing:
Artificial breathing must be started at once, before the victim is completely out of the water, if possible. As soon as the victim's body can be supported, either in a boat or in shallow water, start mouth-to-mouth breathing (see pp. 33–34). Once the victim is out of the water, lay him or her on his or her back on a firm surface and continue mouth-to-mouth resuscitation and CPR if necessary (see p. 30).

If a board is not available:

If the victim is facedown in the water, gently turn him or her over, keeping the head, neck, and body in alignment. Gently tow or push the victim to shallow water and stay with him or her. *Do not* drag the victim sideways. Pull him or her by the armpits or legs in the direction of the length of the body. Keep the head in line with the body. Call for help or have someone get help for you.

If the victim is breathing:

1. Watch the victim to ensure that he or she continues to breathe on his or her own. *Do not* give the victim food or water.
2. Place the victim on his or her side with the head extended backward so that fluids will drain.
3. Keep the victim comfortably warm.
4. Reassure the victim.
5. Seek medical attention promptly.

SHALLOW WATER BLACKOUT

Shallow water blackout is a condition that most often occurs when an individual—usually a child—hyperventilates on purpose in an effort to stay under water for a longer period of time. The process of hyperventilation, however, removes carbon dioxide from the blood, which at normal levels triggers the involuntary stimulus to breathe. Although the individual may actually be capable of staying longer under water, he or she may pass out because of the lack of oxygen.

The condition also results when young, inexperienced divers use 100 percent oxygen rebreather masks in training, usually at depths of 10 to 20 feet. In either situation, the person seldom has a warning before he or she loses consciousness. If not noticed in time, the individual may drown.

SYMPTOMS

- Has been under water, or facedown in the water, longer than usual
- Appears to be lifeless in the water

WHAT TO DO

1. Remove the victim at once from the water.
2. Maintain an open airway. Restore breathing and circulation if necessary, pp. 31–50.
3. Take the victim to the nearest hospital emergency department for further evaluation.

Water Safety

Here are some steps you can take to prevent drowning:

• Never swim alone.
• Don't drink alcohol while swimming or boating.
• Avoid swimming in very cold water (under 82°F).

See Also: Head, Neck, and Back Injuries, p. 194.

INJURIES AND ILLNESSES

Drug abuse is the regular or excessive use of a drug outside the usual standards of medical practice or medical need. Drug abuse often results in physical and psychological dependence on the drug. If you are using drugs, this section will provide you with information about drug overdose and withdrawal and first-aid measures for yourself or for another person. We strongly urge you to see a physician for a confidential discussion about your drug use and information about treatment.

Questions to ask yourself if you suspect that someone you know is using drugs: How is the individual acting differently than normal? Is he or she moody, overly quiet, or easily agitated? Are there physical manifestations that might suggest drug use, such as a sudden loss of weight or an inattention to personal hygiene? Has the individual's group of friends changed within the past 6 months? Do you know who they are? Has the person stopped seeing his or her old friends? Does he or she spend more time alone?

Mild changes in behavior, especially in teenagers, do not necessarily mean that an individual is taking drugs. If you suspect drug use, however, other clues may be helpful in identifying the problem. For example, use of any drug either depresses the central nervous system or stimulates it. Depending on the type of drug and the amount taken, a person's behavior under the influence of that drug may range from extreme sluggishness to hyperactivity. With drugs that are injected into the body, you may notice needle marks on the victim's arms or legs (or elsewhere). In cases of drug withdrawal, you may notice frequent blinking or jerky eye movements, along with the symptoms listed on the following pages.

Paraphernalia that may signal drug use include needles and syringes, eye droppers, teaspoons, pills, capsules, vials, pipes, or glass bulbs ("bongs").

Information to help you recognize the symptoms of drug or alcohol abuse, or withdrawal from dependence on some drugs, is given in the following pages, under categories of drugs. Here are some general guidelines for dealing with drug-related emergencies:

- Professional medical treatment for a person who is suffering withdrawal from drugs or who has overdosed on drugs will vary according to the type of drug and the amount taken.
- For the first-aider faced with an emergency situation in which drug use is suspected, first assess whether or not it is safe for you to handle the situation on your own. If it is not, call out for help.
- If the victim is unconscious, ensure that he or she is breathing. Restore breathing and circulation if necessary. (See pp. 31–50.)
- If the victim is conscious and you are the first person providing first aid, ask the victim what drug he or she took, the amount, and when it was taken. (Report all information, including first-aid treatment, to the doctor later.)

ALCOHOL

Ethanol is the active or "toxic" ingredient in alcoholic beverages that causes intoxication. Alcohol can appear to act as a stimulant but, in fact, is a depressant. It slows down or depresses the activities of the central nervous system (the brain and spinal cord), which controls psychomotor skills such as reaction time and coordination, and areas of the brain that control speech, hearing, and eye movement. Alcohol also impairs reasoning by relaxing an individual's social inhibitions and self-control. Ingesting alcoholic beverages can give a false sense of euphoria.

Alcohol Overdose

SYMPTOMS

Excessive consumption of alcohol can cause any or all of the following symptoms:

- Lack of coordination
- Slurred speech
- Abnormal breathing
- Unconsciousness
- Vomiting
- Coma
- Red streaks in the whites of the eyes
- Odor of alcohol on the breath
- Fast heart rate

INJURIES AND ILLNESSES

- If the victim appears to be sleeping, with normal breathing and pulse, and he or she can be aroused with a shout or a shake, no immediate treatment is required. Place the victim so that he or she will not hurt himself or herself. Check on the victim at regular intervals.
- If the victim has abnormal breathing, is unconscious (cannot be aroused), or is in a coma, maintain an open airway. Restore breathing and circulation if necessary. (See pp. 31–50.) Seek medical attention promptly.

Alcohol Withdrawal

SYMPTOMS

Withdrawal from alcohol dependence can cause any or all of the following symptoms:

- Trembling of hands and head
- Nausea
- Vomiting
- Fear of sounds, ordinary objects, or lights
- Hallucinations (seeing objects that are not present)
- Unusual behavior

WHAT TO DO

1. Seek medical attention promptly.
2. If the victim is vomiting, see that he or she does not choke on vomit.
3. Calm and reassure the victim.

DEPRESSANTS

Depressants are drugs that slow down or depress the activities of the central nervous system (the brain and spinal cord), which controls psychomotor skills such as reaction time and coordination, and areas of the brain that control speech, hearing, eye movement, and perception.

Depressants include all alcoholic beverages, narcotics, sedatives, cannabis drugs, and all depressant tranquilizers. Examples are opium, morphine, heroin, fentanyl (synthetic heroin), codeine, phenobarbital, sleeping pills, marijuana, and hashish. Some of these substances are referred to on the street as weed, downers, goofballs, yellow jackets, red devils, and rainbows.

Depressant Overdose

SYMPTOMS

An overdose of a depressant drug can cause any or all of the following symptoms:

- Intoxicated behavior
- Slurred speech
- Deep sleep, possibly leading to coma
- Shallow breathing

- Slow pulse
- Low body temperature
- Heavy sweating
- Very relaxed muscles
- Very small pupils

WHAT TO DO

1. Call 911 (or your local emergency number). Maintain an open airway. Restore breathing and circulation if necessary. (See pp. 31–50.)
2. Keep the victim awake. Use a cold, wet towel or cloth to slap the victim's face gently.
3. Keep the victim talking, if possible.
4. Calm and reassure the victim.

Depressant Withdrawal

SYMPTOMS

Withdrawal from dependence on depressant drugs can cause any or all of the following symptoms, which may not occur at the same time:

- Nervousness or restlessness
- Trembling
- Muscle twitching
- Abdominal cramping
- Hot and cold flashes
- Sweating
- Weight loss
- Enlarged pupils

- Tears
- Runny nose
- Yawning
- Muscle aches
- Vomiting
- Loss of appetite
- Rise in body temperature
- Craving for the drug

INJURIES AND ILLNESSES

WHAT TO DO

1. Seek medical attention.
2. Calm and reassure the victim.

HALLUCINOGENS

Hallucinogenic drugs, sometimes called psychedelic drugs, change the chemical makeup of the brain and distort perception. The most well-known hallucinogens include lysergic acid diethylamide (LSD or acid), phencyclidine (PCP or angel dust), mescaline and peyote, and psilocybin (magic mushrooms). The effects of hallucinogens can last up to 12 hours. Some stimulants and tetrahydrocannabinol (THC, the active ingredient in marijuana and hashish) can also be hallucinogenic.

Hallucinogen Use

SYMPTOMS

Even one dose of a hallucinogen can cause any or all of the following symptoms:

- Delusions (misinterpretation of sounds, movements, or objects)
- Hallucinations (seeing things that are not present)
- Fast heartbeat
- Increased blood pressure
- Enlarged pupils
- Reddish face
- Lack of emotional control (periods of laughing and crying or behavior not appropriate for the situation)
- Depression (appearing sad or slow to move or talk)
- Panic, fear, or tension
- Varying levels of consciousness
- Disorientation
- Poor recent memory

WHAT TO DO

1. Ensure that the victim does not harm himself or herself or others.
2. Seek medical attention promptly.

3. Reassure the victim and try to talk him or her through the experience in a quiet place.
4. Do not move suddenly in front of the victim. Keep your voice calm and do not turn away from the victim. The victim could try to harm you.

INHALANTS

Increasing numbers of children are inhaling common household products to get high. When used in this way, these substances are called inhalants. Inhalants include glues and adhesives, nail polish remover, marking pens, paint thinner, spray paint, butane lighter fluid, gasoline, propane gas, correction fluid, household cleaners, cooking sprays, deodorants, fabric protectors, whipping cream aerosols, and air-conditioning coolants. These products are usually snorted from a plastic bag or breathed in ("huffed") from a chemical-soaked rag. Using an inhalant even once can damage the brain and nervous system or cause sudden death. While a person is using an inhalant or immediately after, his or her heart may begin to overwork, beating rapidly but unevenly and causing cardiac arrest.

Inhalant Use

SYMPTOMS

Use of inhalants can cause any or all of the following symptoms:

- Intoxicated behavior, loss of coordination, or slurred or disoriented speech
- State of excitement quickly followed by extreme drowsiness
- Hallucinations
- Severe mood swings
- Numbness and tingling of the hands and feet
- Heart palpitations
- Difficulty breathing
- Dizziness
- Red or runny eyes or nose
- Headache
- Death

INJURIES AND ILLNESSES

1. Seek medical attention and intervention immediately.
2. If the person is not breathing, call 911 (or your local emergency number). Maintain an open airway. Restore breathing and circulation if necessary. (See pp. 31–50.)

STIMULANTS

Stimulants increase the activities of the central nervous system (brain and spinal cord), which controls psychomotor skills such as reaction time and coordination, and areas of the brain that control speech, hearing, eye movement, and perception.

Stimulants include amphetamines, cocaine, and inhalants. Some of these substances are referred to on the street as crack, ice (crystal meth), speed, crank, uppers, pep pills, bennies, whites, and dexies.

Stimulant Overdose

SYMPTOMS

An overdose of a stimulant can cause any or all of the following symptoms:

- Overly active behavior
- Aggressive behavior
- Mental confusion
- Disorganization
- Suspiciousness
- Unconsciousness
- Repetition of a particular act
- Irritability
- Fear
- Exaggerated perceptions of personal abilities

WHAT TO DO

1. Approach the victim carefully.
2. Maintain an open airway. Restore breathing and circulation if necessary. (See pp. 31–50.)
3. Seek immediate medical attention.
4. Keep victim from harming himself or herself or others.

Withdrawal

SYMPTOMS

Withdrawal from dependence on stimulants can cause any or all of the following symptoms:

- Extreme lack of energy
- Depression
- Extreme hunger
- Hallucinations
- Deep sleep
- Dehydration

WHAT TO DO

1. Seek medical attention.
2. Calm and reassure the victim.

INJURIES AND ILLNESSES

EAR PROBLEMS

EAR INJURIES

The eardrum can be ruptured by a loud blast, infection, diving, waterskiing falls, objects poked into the ear, or a head injury (such as a slap on the ear). Blood or other fluids coming from the ear canal may indicate a serious head injury. All ear injuries should be considered serious and require medical attention because of the possibility of hearing loss.

SYMPTOMS

An ear injury can cause any or all of the following symptoms:

- Bleeding from inside the ear canal
- Pain
- Hearing loss
- Dizziness

WHAT TO DO

1. If bleeding is due to a head injury with a possible skull fracture, treat the head injury first. The victim should not be moved if a serious head, neck, or back injury is suspected unless his or her life is in danger. (See Head, Neck, and Back Injuries, p. 194.)
2. Loosely cover the outside of the ear with a bandage or cloth to catch the flow of blood. *Do not* try to stop the flow of blood from the ear canal. *Do not* put anything into the ear.
3. Place the victim on his or her injured side with the affected ear down, allowing blood to drain.
4. Seek medical attention promptly.

EARACHES

There are many causes of pain in the ear. One of the most common is an infection of the outer ear caused by a fingernail scratch. Swimming in contaminated water can cause "swimmer's ear." Symptoms of swimmer's ear may include mild pain (particularly when the ear is pulled), itching, and a discharge of water (which has remained in the ear after swimming) from the ear. This condition requires medical attention. Occasionally, ear pain is caused by a medical problem elsewhere in the body, such as a sore throat or temporomandibular joint dysfunction (a condition in which the ligaments, muscles, and joints of the jaw are out of alignment).

Earaches in the middle ear often follow respiratory infections when germs in the nose and throat move through the eustachian tube to the middle ear. Children are particularly susceptible to middle ear infections because their eustachian tubes are shorter than those of adults. Infected tonsils may also cause a middle ear infection. Symptoms of a middle ear infection may include pain, fever, and, rarely, a discharge from the ear. An infant with an ear infection cries loudly, particularly when lying down, pulls or bats at his or her ear, or turns his or her head from side to side. Medical attention is required for treatment of middle ear infections.

NOTE: Never put cotton-tipped swabs, hairpins, matches, or anything else in the ear.

Preventing Swimmer's Ear

Here are some steps you can take to avoid swimmer's ear:

- Do not swim in pools that don't have chlorine.
- After swimming, get the water out of your ears by tilting your head to the side and jumping up and down several times. Do this for both ears. Or dry each ear by blowing a hair dryer into it. Set the dryer at the lowest setting and hold it several inches away from the ear as you gently pull down on the lobe with your other hand.
- When surfing or windsurfing, wear a properly fitted swimming cap or wet suit hood.
- Use silicone earplugs (not wax earplugs) when swimming.

INJURIES AND ILLNESSES

- Ask your doctor about using ear drops or flushing out your ears with an ear syringe and warm water or vinegar after swimming.
- If earwax tends to build up in your ears, you may be susceptible to swimmer's ear; ask your doctor about the best way to keep earwax under control.

FOREIGN OBJECTS INSIDE THE EAR

Children often put objects—such as peas, beans, beads, paper, and cotton balls—in their ears. Insects may also get trapped inside the ear. Most foreign objects lodge in the outer portion of the ear.

WHAT TO DO

1. All small objects trapped inside the ear need medical attention for removal. The only possible exception is paper or cotton if it is clearly visible outside the ear canal. In this instance, you may attempt to remove the object carefully with tweezers. A doctor should be seen, however, to make sure all of it is removed.
2. *Do not* put water or oil into the ear to attempt to flush out the object, unless the object is a live insect (see below). Putting a liquid into the ear could cause the object to swell and make removal more difficult.
3. If an insect inside the ear is alive and buzzing, put several drops of warm oil (such as baby, mineral, or olive oil) into the ear to kill the insect. This is the only time putting oil into the ear is justified. Seek medical attention for removal of the insect.

FROSTBITTEN EARS

Frostbite is freezing of parts of the body from exposure to very low temperatures. Frostbite occurs when ice crystals form in the fluid inside cells of the skin and other tissues. The ears are one of the parts of the body that are affected most often.

SYMPTOMS

Frostbite can cause any or all of the following symptoms:

- Redness and pain (in early stages)
- White or grayish yellow, waxy-looking skin (in later stages)
- Coldness and numbness
- Absence of pain (in later stages)
- Blisters

WARNING

SEVERE FROSTBITE

If severe frostbite has occurred, the victim may not have feeling in his or her ears and the ears may be black, which indicates that skin tissue has died. In this case, cover the ears with warm materials and take the victim without delay to the nearest hospital emergency department for treatment.

WHAT TO DO

1. While outside, cover the ears with extra clothing or a warm cloth. *Do not* rub the ears with snow or anything else.
2. Bring the victim inside promptly.
3. Rewarm the ears rapidly (which may cause pain). Gently wrap the ears for 15 to 30 minutes in warm materials, such as moist, warm compresses or dry towels heated in an oven to 100°F to 104°F. Or place the palms of your hands over the victim's ears. *Do not* use heat lamps, hot water bottles, or heating pads and *do not* allow the victim to place frostbitten ears near a hot stove or radiator (frostbitten parts could be burned because of the lack of pain sensation).
4. Stop the warming process when the skin becomes pink. *Do not* break any blisters. Blisters are a natural barrier against infection.
5. Give the victim warm drinks such as tea, coffee, or soup. *Do not* give the victim alcoholic beverages (alcohol restricts the blood flow).
6. Seek medical attention promptly.
7. Take extreme care that frostbitten ears are not exposed to cold before they have thawed completely.

INJURIES AND ILLNESSES

ELECTRICAL BURNS

Electrical burns may appear slight on the surface of the skin, but can be extremely severe in the underlying tissue. Exposure to ordinary household electrical current seldom causes serious problems, but exposure to high-voltage wires is usually fatal.

If you are the first person offering first aid to the victim of an electrical burn, it is extremely important not to risk electrocuting yourself. *Do not* touch the victim directly until the electric current is turned off or the victim is no longer in contact with it. Victims who have been struck by lightning may be touched immediately because they are no longer connected to a continuous supply of electricity.

All electrical burns, no matter how minor they may seem, require immediate medical attention.

SYMPTOMS

Electrical burns can cause any or all of the following symptoms:

- Slight redness at the site of the burn
- Muscle spasm

WHAT TO DO

1. If possible, turn off the electric current by removing the fuse or by pulling the main switch. If this is not possible, or if the victim is outside, have someone call the electric company to cut off the electricity. Try to stay at least 60 feet away from a high-voltage line.
2. If it is necessary to remove the victim from a live wire, be extremely careful. Stand on something dry, such as a newspaper, board, blanket, rubber mat, or cloth, and, if possible, wear dry gloves. Push the victim away from the wire with a dry board, stick, broom handle, or well-insulated wooden tool, or pull the

victim away with a dry rope looped around the victim's arm or leg. Never use anything metallic, wet, or damp. Do not touch the victim until he or she is free from the wire.

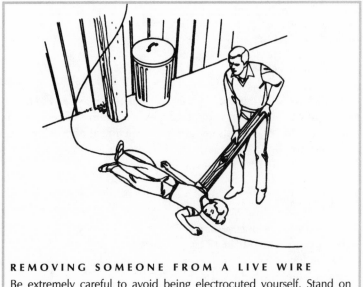

REMOVING SOMEONE FROM A LIVE WIRE
Be extremely careful to avoid being electrocuted yourself. Stand on something dry, wear dry gloves if possible, and push the victim away from the wire with a dry board, stick, or tool—or pull the victim away with a dry rope looped around the victim's arm or leg.

3. If the victim is not breathing, call 911 (or your local emergency number). Maintain an open airway. Restore breathing and circulation if necessary. (See pp. 31–50.)
4. Cover the burn with a clean, dry dressing. Be careful not to break any blisters.
5. Look for signs of broken bones or neck injuries from a fall.
6. Seek immediate medical attention no matter how minor the burn may seem.

CHEMICAL BURNS

Chemical burns of the eye are very serious and may lead to blindness if immediate action is not taken. Acids, drain cleaner, bleach, and other cleaning solutions are some chemical agents that can burn the eye. Speed in removing a chemical agent is vital. Damage can occur in 1 to 5 minutes.

WHAT TO DO

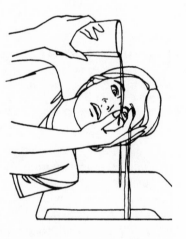

- Before calling a doctor, have the victim remove his or her contact lenses and then immediately flush the eye with large quantities of cool, running water for at least 10 minutes to rinse out the chemical agent. Use milk if water is not available. Hold the victim's head under a faucet (or shower, hose, or pitcher of water), with the eyelids held open, and allow the water to run from the inside corner (next to the nose) outward so that the water flows over the entire eye and so that the chemical does not get in the unaffected eye. If both eyes are affected, let water flow over both or quickly alternate between one eye and the other. Be sure to lift and separate the eyelids so the water reaches all parts of the eye.
- Another method is to place the top of the victim's face in a bowl or sink filled with water with the eyes in the water, and have the victim move the eyelids up and down.

- If the victim is lying down, pour large quantities of water from a container from the inside corner of the eye outward, keeping the eyelids open. Keep repeating this procedure.
- After following one of the above steps, cover the injured eye or eyes with a pad of sterile gauze or a clean folded handkerchief, and tape it in place with the eyelids closed.
- *Do not* allow the victim to rub the eyes.
- Seek medical attention immediately, preferably at the nearest hospital emergency department.

BLOWS TO THE EYE

Any injury resulting from a hard, direct blow to the eye, such as from a moving ball or a fist, needs medical attention by an ophthalmologist even though the injury may not look serious. There may be internal bleeding in the eye. A black eye usually takes 2 to 3 weeks to clear up.

WHAT TO DO

1. If the victim is wearing contact lenses, do not remove them; a physician should remove them as soon as possible.
2. Apply cold compresses to the injured eye.
3. If possible, keep the victim lying down with eyes closed and head elevated.
4. Seek immediate medical attention.

WARNING

SUDDEN EYE PAIN OR BLURRED VISION

Any sudden pain in the eyes without recent injury or a sudden blurring or loss of vision requires immediate medical attention.

INJURIES AND ILLNESSES

EYE INFECTIONS

Chalazion

A chalazion is an infection and inflammation of a deep gland in the underside of the eyelid.

SYMPTOMS

- Round, painless bump (in early stages)
- Hard, red, painful bump (in later stages)
- Blurred vision

WHAT TO DO

1. Have the victim remove his or her contact lenses.
2. Apply warm water compresses to the outer eyelid several times a day. Do not try to "pop" the bump.
3. If the bump persists for several days or recurs, seek medical attention.

Conjunctivitis

Conjunctivitis (sometimes referred to as pinkeye) is an infection of the eye that is usually caused by fungi, bacteria, allergies, or chemicals. The infection may affect one or both eyes. Certain forms of conjunctivitis can be very contagious for several days.

SYMPTOMS

Conjunctivitis can cause any or all of the following symptoms:

- Redness of the white portion of the eye
- Watery or sticky, yellow, green, or brown discharge from the eye
- Sticky upper and lower eyelashes, particularly in the morning
- Sensation of something in the eye

WHAT TO DO

1. Have the victim remove his or her contact lenses.
2. Consult a physician.

3. Place an ice cube in a plastic bag and hold it over the eyelid for temporary relief of pain.
4. Wash your hands (and towels and washcloths) after any contact with the infected eye.

Stye

A stye is an inflammation of the glands of the edge of the eyelid.

SYMPTOMS

A stye can cause any or all of the following symptoms:

• Tender, red, pimplelike bumps near the edge of the eyelid
• Itching or tearing

WHAT TO DO

1. Have the victim remove his or her contact lenses.
2. Apply warm water compresses to the affected area several times a day. *Do not* try to "pop" the stye.
3. If the stye persists for several days or recurs, seek medical attention.

CUTS

Any cuts to the eye, including the eyelid, can be very serious and could lead to blindness if immediate action is not taken.

WHAT TO DO

1. If the victim is wearing contact lenses, do not remove them; a physician should remove them as soon as possible.
2. Gently cover *both* eyes (because when one moves, so does the other) with a sterile pad or gauze or a clean folded cloth and tape it lightly in place without applying any pressure.
3. Seek medical attention immediately, preferably from an eye specialist (such as an ophthalmologist) or at the nearest hospital emergency department. Transport the victim lying down flat on his or her back if possible.

INJURIES AND ILLNESSES

173

FOREIGN OBJECTS IN THE EYE

Never attempt to remove any particle that is sticking out of the eyeball. Seek immediate medical attention for such injuries. Particles such as eyelashes, cinders, or specks that are resting or floating on the eyeball or inside the eyelid may be carefully removed.

SYMPTOMS

A foreign object in the eye can cause any or all of the following symptoms:

- Pain
- Burning sensation
- Tearing
- Redness of the eye
- Sensitivity to light

WHAT TO DO

If the foreign object is embedded in the eye:

1. Wash your hands with soap and water before carefully examining the victim's eyes. *Do not* allow the victim to rub his or her eyes or to remove his or her contact lenses.
2. If you can see that the foreign object is embedded in the eyeball, *do not* attempt to remove the object.
3. Gently cover *both* eyes (because when one moves, so does the other) with a sterile compress and tape it lightly in place without applying any pressure. If compresses are not available, use a scarf, a large cloth napkin, or other suitable material and tie it around the victim's head.
4. Seek medical attention promptly, preferably from an ophthalmologist or at the nearest hospital emergency department. Keep the victim lying down on his or her back while riding to the hospital. Use a stretcher if possible.

If the foreign object is resting or floating on the eye or inside the eyelid:

1. Wash your hands with soap and water before carefully examining the victim's eyes. *Do not* allow the victim to rub his or her eyes or to remove his or her contact lenses.

2. Gently pull the upper eyelid down over the lower eyelid and hold for a moment. This causes tears to flow, which may wash out the particle.

3. If the particle has not been removed, fill a medicine dropper with warm water and squeeze water over the eye to flush out the particle. If a medicine dropper is not available, hold the victim's head under a gentle stream of running water, or use a glass of water, to flush out the particle.

4. If still unsuccessful, gently pull the lower eyelid down. If the foreign object can be seen on the inside of the lower lid, carefully lift the particle out with a moistened, clean cloth or tissue.

REMOVING A PARTICLE FROM THE EYE

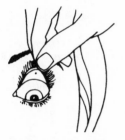

To remove a particle resting on the inside of the upper lid, have the person look down as you hold the lashes of the upper eyelid and pull the eyelid upward.

While holding the eyelid place a cotton-tipped swab across the back of the lid and flip the eyelid backward over it.

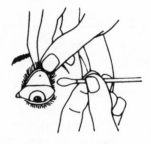

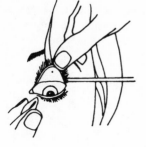

Carefully remove the particle with a moistened, clean cloth or tissue.

5. If the speck is not visible on the lower lid, check the inside of the upper lid by holding the lashes of the upper eyelid and pulling downward. The person must look down during the entire procedure. While holding the eyelid down, place a cotton-tipped swab across the back of the lid and flip the eyelid backward over it. (The person can help by holding the swab.) Carefully remove the particle with a moistened, clean cloth or tissue.

6. If the particle still remains, gently cover the eye with a sterile or clean compress and seek medical attention promptly.

GLUE ON THE EYELIDS

When working with glue, people sometimes transfer glue from their hands to their eyelids, causing the eyelids to stick together.

WHAT TO DO

• If the eyelids are completely stuck together, never try to pull them apart. Seek medical attention promptly.
• If the eyelids are partially stuck together, rinse them with water to loosen the glue. Seek medical attention promptly.

SUNBURN OF THE EYE

The eyes—especially the protective, transparent coating over the front of the eye (the cornea)—are extremely sensitive to damage from ultraviolet rays from the sun. These burns, often referred to as snow blindness, are most likely to occur at high altitudes when a thick coating of snow is on the ground (skiers and mountain climbers are especially susceptible). People who use tanning salons are also at risk of eye burns. The best way to prevent burns of the eyes or the eyelids is to wear sunglasses that have attached side panels and to apply sunscreen to the eyelids before going out in the sun.

SYMPTOMS

Sunburn of the eyes can cause any or all of the following symptoms, which usually occur within 12 hours of exposure:

- Redness of the eye
- Severe pain, especially in light (but vision is usually not affected)
- Spasm of the eyelids

WHAT TO DO

1. Avoid sunlight.
2. Seek medical attention promptly.

INJURIES AND ILLNESSES

FAINTING

Fainting is a brief loss of consciousness due to a reduced blood supply reaching the brain. Recovery usually occurs within a few minutes. Fainting sometimes occurs during the first 5 days of exposure to hot weather, before a person's body becomes adapted to the heat. People who are taking diuretics are at increased risk of fainting in hot weather.

SYMPTOMS

Fainting may be preceded by any or all of the following symptoms:

- Pale, cool, and wet skin
- Light-headedness or dizziness
- Nausea
- Feeling of restlessness
- Frequent yawning

WHAT TO DO

If the person is about to faint or feels faint:
1. Have the person lie down with legs elevated 8 to 12 inches, or have him or her sit down and slowly bend the body forward so that his or her head is between the knees.
2. Move any harmful objects out of the way and calm and reassure the person.
3. If you suspect the person's condition may be caused by hot weather, assist him or her to a cooler place. Encourage him or her to drink plenty of fluids to prevent dehydration.

If the person has fainted and is not breathing:
1. Call 911 (or your local emergency number).
2. Maintain an open airway. Restore breathing and circulation if necessary. (See pp. 31–50.)

If the person has fainted and is breathing:
1. If you suspect that the fainting may have been caused by hot weather, move the person to a cooler place. Encourage him or her to drink plenty of fluids to prevent dehydration.
2. Keep the person lying down. Elevate his or her feet 8 to 12 inches (unless the person has fallen and a head injury is suspected).
3. Maintain an open airway.
4. Loosen tight clothing, particularly around the neck. *Do not* give the person anything to drink unless he or she seems fully recovered.
5. If the person vomits, place him or her on his or her side. Or, turn the head sideways to prevent choking on vomit.
6. Gently bathe the person's face with cool water. *Do not* pour water on the face.
7. Check for injuries that may have been caused by falling.
8. Observe the person after he or she regains consciousness. Calm and reassure him or her.
9. If recovery does not seem complete within a few minutes, seek medical attention.

INJURIES AND ILLNESSES

A fever is the body's way of indicating that something is wrong—most commonly that an infection is present. A fever is the body's defensive mechanism to combat infection. You should always call a doctor if a fever suddenly changes from slight (99°F to 100°F) to high (104°F) and persists. If the person with a fever is an infant and a doctor cannot be reached, take the child to the nearest hospital emergency department. The same steps should be taken if a fever is present for no obvious reason and it persists. In this case, it is best not to take any medication to reduce the fever, as this may give the person a false sense of well-being and discourage him or her from consulting a doctor.

FEVER IN ADULTS

The average normal temperature taken by mouth is 98.6°F, plus or minus 1°. A rectal temperature is 1° higher than a normal oral temperature. Individual normal temperatures may run slightly above or below the average. Individual temperatures may also vary throughout the day, running lower in the morning and higher in the evening. Slight changes in temperature (other than normal variations during the day) are usually not significant. A major increase in temperature (to approximately 104°F or over) may indicate a serious condition. Temperatures well below normal may also be significant.

WHAT TO DO

Take aspirin or a nonsteroidal anti-inflammatory medication such as ibuprofen, acetaminophen, or naproxen to help reduce the fever. Follow the package recommendations or a doctor's instructions to determine the dose to take. Remove excess clothing and move the person to a cooler environment.

FEVER IN INFANTS AND CHILDREN

A normal temperature taken rectally in infants and small children is usually below 100°F. Rectal temperature readings run about 1° higher than oral temperature readings. Although temperature is the same throughout the body, taking an oral temperature lets air into the mouth, lowering the temperature reading somewhat. Children can run high fevers without being seriously ill. It is always best, however, to report any fever over 101°F to the doctor, particularly if the child does not feel, look, or act well. Report to the doctor any other symptoms the child might have.

WARNING

DON'T GIVE ASPIRIN TO CHILDREN

Never give aspirin to a child under 18 years. The use of aspirin in children has been linked to a life-threatening disorder called Reye's syndrome.

WHAT TO DO

1. Always check with the doctor before giving medication to an infant or small child, particularly one under 1 year of age.
2. Give the child plenty of fluids.
3. Have the child rest in bed if possible.
4. Reduce a high fever (104°F or over) by sponging the child with warm water and letting the water evaporate on the skin. Recheck the temperature every 25 to 30 minutes. Continue giving sponge baths until rectal temperature is below 102°F. Be careful that the child does not become chilled.

INJURIES AND ILLNESSES

FINGERTIP INJURIES

Injuries to the fingertip resulting from a hammer hit or slammed door are extremely painful. Small blood vessels under the fingernail may break, causing a blood clot to form. Within 1 to 2 days, the nail turns black. The area becomes very painful from the pressure of the blood clot.

It is recommended that a doctor remove the blood clot, especially if it is deep beneath the fingernail. However, if medical assistance is not available for a few days and the pain is severe, drain the blood clot yourself by following these instructions:

WHAT TO DO

1. Sterilize a needle or paper clip (straightened out) by holding it over an open flame until it is red hot.
2. Gently puncture the blood clot to allow it to drain by pushing the needle or paper clip through the fingernail into the clot area. You may have to puncture the clot several times in order to drain it.
3. Cover the area with a sterile bandage. The fingernail should not be pulled off if it becomes loose. Keep the nail in place with a bandage to allow the new fingernail to push off the old one.
4. If the pain is not relieved immediately or it gets worse, or if the clot is as large as half the nail, see a physician right away.

FISHHOOK INJURIES

A fishhook caught in the body is a common injury. If the fishhook goes deep enough so that the barb is embedded in the skin, it is best to have a doctor remove it because it may have penetrated bone. If a doctor is not readily available, the hook should be removed.

> **WARNING**
>
> FISHHOOK IN THE EYE OR ON THE FACE
>
> Never attempt to remove a fishhook caught in the eye or face. Seek medical help immediately. If a fishhook is in an eye, have the person hold a cup (preferably a metal one, which won't break or crush) over the eye until you reach the nearest hospital emergency department.

WHAT TO DO

If only the point of the hook (and not the barb) entered the skin, remove the hook by carefully pulling it out.

If the hook is embedded in the skin:

1. Push the hook through the skin until the barb comes out.
2. Cut the hook with pliers or clippers at either the barb or the shank of the hook. Remove the remaining part. For either type of injury, clean the wound with soap and water, cover with a bandage, and seek medical attention as soon as possible. There is always the possibility of infection and the need for a tetanus shot.

REMOVING A FISHHOOK

The fishhook is embedded beyond the barb in the tip of the finger.

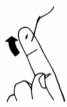

To remove it, push the hook through the skin until the barb comes out.

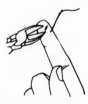

Cut the hook with pliers or clippers at the barb or at the shank.

Carefully remove the remaining part of the hook.

Suspect food poisoning if several people become ill with similar symptoms at approximately the same time after eating the same food. Also suspect food poisoning if one person becomes ill after eating food no one else has eaten.

BOTULISM

Botulism is a very serious form of food poisoning that is often fatal. It is a medical emergency. Botulism most often occurs after eating improperly home-canned foods but some cases have occurred after eating commercially prepared frozen foods, including pot pies, asparagus, green beans, peppers, and onions sautéed with margarine. Botulism has also been associated with eating some seafood, including salmon or seal, walrus, or whale meat.

SYMPTOMS

Botulism can cause any or all of the following symptoms, which usually appear within 6 to 72 hours:

- Dry mouth
- Dizziness
- Headache
- Blurred and/or double vision
- Muscle weakness
- Difficulty swallowing
- Difficulty talking
- Difficulty breathing
- Hoarseness
- Incoordination

WHAT TO DO

Seek medical attention immediately, preferably at the nearest hospital emergency department.

> ### Preventing Botulism
>
> Here are some steps you can take to avoid botulism:
>
> • Do not keep cooked foods at room temperature (or higher than 40°F) for longer than 2 hours.
> • Freeze foods for long-term storage.
> • Discard cans that have defects such as swelling.
> • When preserving foods, boil them for at least 10 minutes at a temperature higher than 212°F. (Dry-heating methods such as smoking do not kill the botulism toxin.) Use proper preserving techniques such as high acidity or nitrate preservatives.

CAMPYLOBACTER POISONING

Food poisoning caused by the campylobacter bacterium is becoming increasingly common. Most cases occur during the summer. The bacterium is found in undercooked poultry, raw milk, and polluted water.

SYMPTOMS

Campylobacter poisoning can cause any or all of the following symptoms, which usually appear within 4 days of eating the contaminated food and last about 1 week:

• Diarrhea (sometimes with blood)
• Abdominal cramps
• Nausea and vomiting
• Headache
• Fever

WHAT TO DO

1. Keep the person lying down and comfortably warm.
2. After the person has stopped vomiting, give him or her warm, mild fluids such as tea, broth, or fruit juice.
3. Seek medical attention promptly.

COCCIDIAN PARASITE INFECTIONS

Coccidian parasites, *Cryptosporidium parvum* and *Cyclospora cayetanensis,* are microorganisms that have been associated with unpasteurized apple cider, raw vegetables and fruits, and contaminated water. Infection with either of these parasites can cause severe, prolonged watery diarrhea.

SYMPTOMS

Food poisoning from coccidian parasites can cause any or all of the following symptoms, which usually start 3 to 9 days after eating contaminated food and can last up to a month:

- Severe, watery diarrhea
- Fever and chills
- Headache
- Body aches
- Abdominal cramps
- Nausea and/or vomiting

WHAT TO DO

1. Keep the person lying down and comfortably warm.
2. After the person has stopped vomiting, give him or her warm, mild fluids such as tea, broth, or fruit juice.
3. Seek medical attention promptly.

E. COLI INFECTIONS

A dangerous form of the *E. coli* (short for *Escherichia coli*) bacterium, called *E. coli* O157:H7, can cause severe, bloody diarrhea that can be fatal. Infection with this bacterium has been associated primarily with eating contaminated ground beef. Other sources include unpasteurized milk and milk products and unpasteurized fruit juice. Some outbreaks have been linked to contaminated sand, soil, modeling clay, and leaking of a soiled diaper into a swimming pool. Severe infections with *E. coli* O157:H7 can damage the kidneys, heart, lungs, and central nervous system. Children under 5 years and the elderly are at highest risk of having a severe infection.

INJURIES AND ILLNESSES

SYMPTOMS

Infection with *E. coli* O157:H7 can cause any or all of the following symptoms:

- Bloody diarrhea
- Abdominal cramps

WHAT TO DO

1. Keep the person lying down and comfortably warm.
2. After the person has stopped vomiting, give him or her warm, mild fluids such as tea, broth, or fruit juice.
3. Seek medical attention promptly.

Preventing *E. coli* Infections

Here are some steps you can take to avoid infection with *E. coli:*

- Always wash your hands before preparing food, and wash all foods you are going to eat raw.
- After handling raw meat, wash your hands, cutting boards, and any plates, bowls, or utensils the meat came into contact with. Cook all meat and poultry thoroughly.
- Peel fruits and vegetables such as apples and potatoes. Remove the outer layers of leafy vegetables such as lettuce. Rinse fruits and vegetables thoroughly under running water for a minute or two.
- When eating out, do not order rare meat—especially hamburgers and beef.
- Avoid unpasteurized milk products and fruit juices.
- Don't drink unchlorinated water.
- Don't allow a child in diapers to go in a swimming pool and don't allow a child with diarrhea to swim in a pool.
- Never swallow lake water while swimming.

MUSHROOM POISONING

Mushroom poisoning occurs after eating poisonous mushrooms found growing wild.

SYMPTOMS

Mushroom poisoning can cause any or all of the following symptoms, which appear within minutes to 24 hours, depending on the type and amount of mushroom eaten (symptoms may also vary according to the type of mushroom eaten):

- Abdominal pain
- Diarrhea (may contain blood)
- Vomiting (may contain blood)
- Difficulty breathing
- Sweating
- Salivation
- Tears
- Dizziness
- Hallucinations
- Seizures
- Muscle spasms

WHAT TO DO

1. Call the poison control center, hospital emergency department, a doctor, or 911 (or your local emergency number) for instructions.
2. Keep the victim resting in a quiet place.
3. If medical advice is not readily available, induce vomiting if the victim has not already vomited. Vomiting may be induced by giving an adult or child over 12 years old (unless of low weight) 2 tablespoons of syrup of ipecac; a child between the ages of 1 and 11 years, 1 tablespoon; and an infant under 1 year, 2 teaspoons. Follow with one to two glasses of water or milk. If vomiting does not occur within 15 to 20 minutes, repeat the dosage of ipecac only once. *Do not* give mustard or table salt to the victim to induce vomiting.
4. If vomiting occurs, keep the victim facedown, head lower than the rest of the body so that he or she will not choke on the vomit. Place a small child facedown across your knees.
5. Seek medical attention immediately.

SALMONELLA POISONING

Salmonella poisoning usually occurs during the summer after eating fresh food that has been contaminated with salmonella bacteria. Foods most commonly affected include eggs, milk, raw meats, raw poultry, and raw fish. Salmonella poisoning can be very seri-

INJURIES AND ILLNESSES

ous in infants, young children, the elderly, and the chronically ill. Salmonella can be destroyed by heating foods properly.

SYMPTOMS

Salmonella poisoning can cause any or all of the following symptoms, which usually appear from 6 to 24 hours after eating the contaminated food and last 3 to 5 days:

- Abdominal cramps
- Diarrhea
- Fever
- Chills
- Headache

- Vomiting
- Weakness
- Foul-smelling stool
- Watery, green stool with mucus or blood

WHAT TO DO

1. Keep the person lying down and comfortably warm.
2. After the person has stopped vomiting, give him or her warm, mild fluids such as tea, broth, or fruit juice.
3. Seek medical attention promptly.

Preventing Food Poisoning From Eggs

Here are some steps you can take to avoid food poisoning from eggs (usually caused by salmonella or staphylococcal bacteria):

- Eat only pasteurized eggs.
- Keep eggs refrigerated until you cook them.
- Never eat raw eggs.
- Boil eggs for at least 7 minutes.
- Poach eggs for at least 5 minutes.
- Fry eggs on each side for 3 minutes.
- Do not keep incompletely cooked eggs at room temperature for longer than 2 hours.
- Rinse hard-boiled eggs in water that is warmer than the egg itself.

SHIGELLA POISONING

Shigella poisoning is a highly infectious form of diarrhea that usually occurs in children who have been exposed to contaminated food. The foods most likely to be contaminated with shigella bacteria include potatoes, milk products, meat salads, and polluted water. The bacterium can be destroyed by properly heating foods. However, shigella can survive being frozen and thawed.

SYMPTOMS

Shigella poisoning can cause any or all of the following symptoms, which appear from 1 to 3 days after eating the contaminated food and usually subside within a week:

- Abdominal cramps
- Diarrhea
- Foul-smelling stool
- Watery, green stool with mucus or blood
- Chills
- Headache
- Vomiting
- Weakness
- Fever

WHAT TO DO

1. Keep the person lying down and comfortably warm.
2. After the person has stopped vomiting, give him or her warm, mild fluids such as tea, broth, or fruit juice.
3. Seek medical attention promptly.

STAPHYLOCOCCUS POISONING

Staphylococcus poisoning occurs most often by eating foods that have not been properly refrigerated. The most common foods affected include meats, poultry, eggs, milk, cream-filled bakery goods, salami, sausage, ham, tongue, and tuna and potato salad.

INJURIES AND ILLNESSES

SYMPTOMS

Staphylococcus poisoning can cause any or all of the following symptoms, which usually appear 2 to 6 hours after eating the contaminated food and last about a day:

- Abdominal cramps
- Nausea
- Vomiting
- Diarrhea

WHAT TO DO

1. Keep the victim resting, preferably in bed.
2. After vomiting is over, give the victim warm, mild fluids such as tea, broth, or fruit juice.
3. Seek medical attention if the symptoms are severe or persist.

TRAVELER'S DIARRHEA

Traveler's diarrhea is a form of food poisoning that can result from exposure to one of several different bacteria (usually *E. coli,* salmonella, or shigella), viruses, or parasites. The infection occurs most often during the rainy summer months in tropical regions of Africa, Latin America, the Caribbean, southern Asia, and Mediterranean countries.

SYMPTOMS

Traveler's diarrhea can cause any or all of the following symptoms, which usually appear quickly after eating the contaminated food and last up to 3 days:

- Abdominal cramps
- Fever
- Nausea and vomiting
- Watery diarrhea (two to four bowel movements a day)

WHAT TO DO

1. Keep the person lying down and comfortably warm.
2. When the person has stopped vomiting, give him or her warm, mild fluids such as tea, broth, or fruit juice.

3. If the diarrhea is mild and the victim does not have a fever, or if the person has only had vomiting, give 2 tablespoons or two tablets of bismuth subsalicylate every 30 minutes (for an adult)—up to a total of eight doses in all. The medication should not be taken for more than 2 days. Another over-the-counter medication called loperamide can also be taken; give up to 8 milligrams of loperamide a day for no more than 2 days. Talk to your doctor before giving any medication to a child.
4. If the symptoms last longer than 3 days or get worse, seek medical attention.

Preventing Traveler's Diarrhea

Here are some steps you can take to avoid traveler's diarrhea:

- Avoid drinking tap water or ice made from untreated water. Limit your beverages to bottled water, carbonated drinks, beer, or wine.
- Avoid unpasteurized or unrefrigerated milk products or fruit juices.
- Avoid raw vegetables, salads, seafood, and meat.
- Peel all fruits and cook all food to steaming hot. (Dry foods such as bread are probably safe to eat.)
- Ask your doctor about taking medication to prevent traveler's diarrhea. He or she may recommend taking two tablets of bismuth subsalicylate four times a day, starting the day before you leave for your trip and every day during the trip. Bismuth subsalicylate should not be given to children under 5 years or to people who are allergic to aspirin.

See Also: Dehydration, p. 145; Diarrhea, p. 148; Unconsciousness, p. 259; Vomiting, p. 262.

INJURIES AND ILLNESSES

HEAD, NECK, AND
BACK INJURIES

All head injuries must be taken seriously, as they can result in brain or spinal cord damage or even death. Any victim who is found unconscious must be assumed to have a head injury until medical personnel determine otherwise. Most head injuries are caused by a fall, a blow to the head, a collision, or stopping suddenly, as in an automobile collision. Anyone with a head injury may also have a neck injury.

SYMPTOMS

Head injuries may involve any or all of the following symptoms, some of which may not occur immediately:

- Cut, bruise, lump, or depression in the scalp
- Unconsciousness, confusion, or drowsiness
- Bleeding from the nose, ear, or mouth
- Clear or bloody fluid from the nose or ears
- Pale or reddish face
- Headache
- Vomiting
- Convulsions
- Pupils of unequal size
- Difficulty speaking
- Restlessness or confused behavior
- Change in pulse rate

WHAT TO DO

1. Maintain an open airway. Be very careful, as there may be a possibility of a broken neck. Restore breathing if necessary by mouth-to-mouth resuscitation. (See pp. 31–50.)

2. Keep the victim lying down, quiet, and comfortably warm. If you must move the victim, handle him or her very carefully.
3. *Do not* give the victim anything by mouth.
4. Control serious bleeding. (See Bleeding, p. 96.) Gently apply a compress to the bleeding area and tape it in place.
5. Note the length and extent of unusual behavior or unconsciousness.
6. Seek medical attention promptly, preferably at the nearest hospital emergency department. If someone other than trained medical personnel must take the victim to the hospital, transport him or her lying down, *face up*. Place pads or other suitable material on each side of the victim's head to keep it from moving from side to side.

WARNING

DELAYED SYMPTOMS

All head injuries require prompt medical attention, particularly if the victim was or is unconscious. However, if the victim did not lose consciousness at the time of the injury and did not receive medical care, watch closely for delayed symptoms of brain damage for several days. If you notice any of the symptoms of brain damage—particularly unconsciousness, change in pulse, difficulty breathing, convulsions, severe vomiting, pupils of unequal size, or a generally poor or ill appearance—seek medical attention promptly.

INJURIES AND ILLNESSES

WARNING

REMOVING A HELMET

After an accident involving a person who is wearing a helmet, you should not try to remove the helmet because doing so could cause harm. You can sometimes remove the face guard with a screwdriver without risking further injury. Remove the helmet only if the person is having trouble breathing or has stopped breathing and requires CPR, if the person's neck needs to be stabilized, or if the person has severe bleeding from the head. In any of these situations, call 911 (or your local emergency number) first and then carefully remove the helmet following the steps below (note that this procedure requires at least two people):

1. Facing the top of the victim's head, place your hands on each side of the helmet, with your fingers on the victim's lower jaw to immobilize the head.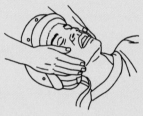
2. Have another person immobilize the victim's head from below by applying pressure to the jaw with the thumb and fingers of one hand and pressure to the base of the skull with the other hand. The hands must hold the head immobile until the helmet is completely removed.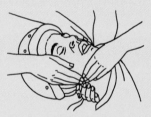
3. Stretch out the sides of the helmet as much as you can and gently and carefully remove it.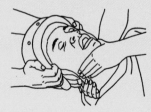

4. Keep the victim's head immobilized from above by placing
your hands on both sides of
the head, with your palms
over the ears. CPR can now
be administered if necessary.
(See p. 30.)

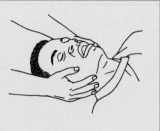

NECK INJURIES

A neck injury should be suspected if a head injury has occurred.
Never move a victim with a suspected neck injury without trained
medical assistance unless the victim is in imminent danger of
death (such as from fire, an explosion, or a collapsing building).

WARNING

KEEP THE HEAD IMMOBILE

Any movement of the head of a person with a neck injury—
either forward, backward, or from side to side—can result in
paralysis or death.

SYMPTOMS

A neck injury may involve any or all of the following symptoms:

• Headache
• Stiff neck
• Inability to move any part of the body
• Inability to move specific parts of the body (such as arms or
  legs)
• Tingling sensation in feet and hands

WHAT TO DO

**If the victim must be moved because of immediate danger to his
or her life:**

INJURIES AND ILLNESSES

1. Immobilize the neck with a rolled towel or newspaper about 4 inches wide wrapped around the neck and tied loosely in place. (*Do not* allow the tie to interfere with the victim's breathing.) If the victim is being rescued from an automobile or from water, place a reasonably short, wide board behind the victim's head and back. The board should extend at least to the buttocks. If possible, tie the board to the victim's body around the forehead and under the armpits. Move the victim very slowly and gently. *Do not* let the victim's body bend or twist.
2. If the victim is not breathing or is having great difficulty breathing, tilt his or her head *slightly* backward to provide and maintain an open airway. Restore breathing and circulation if necessary. (See pp. 31–50.)
3. Call 911 (or your local emergency number) immediately.
4. Lay folded towels, blankets, clothing, sandbags, or other suitable objects around the victim's head, neck, and shoulders to keep the head and neck from moving. Place bricks or stones next to the blankets for additional support.
5. Keep the victim comfortably warm while waiting for medical help to arrive.

If the victim must be taken to the hospital by someone other than trained medical personnel:
1. The victim must be transported lying down on his or her back *face up,* unless there is danger of vomiting, in which case the victim's entire body must be rolled together onto a side, keeping the head in the same line with the body in which it was found.
2. Place a well-padded, rigid support such as a door, table leaf, or wide board next to the victim. Gather something suitable for tying the victim to the board (such as rope, neckties tied together, or strips of strong cloth) and slide them underneath the board in three or four places.
3. If the victim is breathing on his or her own, hold the victim's head in the same line with the body in which it was found. Other helpers should grasp the victim's clothes and *slide* the victim onto the support, moving the entire body together as a unit.
4. Place folded towels, blankets, or cloths around the victim's head and neck to keep them from moving and, if possible, tie the victim's body to the support.

5. Gently lift the board into the transporting vehicle.

6. Drive carefully to the hospital to prevent further injury.

NOTE: If a pregnant woman who has had a head, neck, or back injury needs to be transported to a hospital by someone other than trained medical personnel, have her lie on her left side; this position improves blood flow to the fetus.

IMMOBILIZING A BROKEN NECK

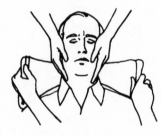

Carefully wrap a towel, sweater, newspaper, or some other cushioned item, about 4 inches wide, around the victim's neck, keeping the head as still as possible.

Tie the wrap in place, being careful not to interfere with the victim's breathing.

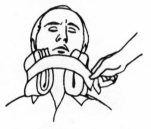

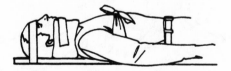

If the victim is being rescued from an automobile or from water, place a board behind the victim's head and back. The board should extend at least to the victim's buttocks. If possible, tie the board to the victim's body around the forehead and under the armpits. Move the victim slowly and gently.

MOVING A VICTIM WITH A HEAD, NECK, OR BACK INJURY

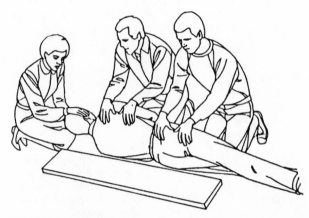

If the victim of a suspected head, neck, or back injury must be taken to the hospital by someone other than trained medical personnel, he or she must be transported lying down. Place a well-padded rigid support, such as a door or table leaf, next to the victim. The support should extend from beyond the head at least to the buttocks.

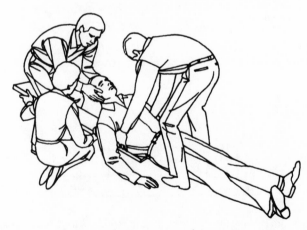

The victim's head must be held so that it stays in the same line with the body in which it was found. Helpers should grasp the victim's clothes and *slide* him or her onto the support. Move the entire body as a unit.

BACK INJURIES

Never move a victim with a suspected back injury without trained medical assistance unless the victim is in immediate danger from fire, an explosion, or any other life-threatening situation. Any movement of the head, neck, or back may result in paralysis or death. With a severe back or neck injury, the victim may not be able to move the arms, hands, fingers, legs, feet, or toes. The victim may also have tingling, numbness, or pain in the neck or back or down the arms or legs.

SYMPTOMS

Severe back injuries can cause any or all of the following symptoms and require immediate medical attention:

- Inability to move the arms, fingers, legs, feet, or toes
- Tingling, numbness, or pain in the neck, back, or down the arms or legs.

WHAT TO DO

1. Call 911 (or your local emergency number).
2. Place folded blankets, towels, or clothing at the victim's sides, head, and neck to keep him or her from rotating or moving from side to side.
3. Keep the victim comfortably warm while waiting for medical help to arrive.

If the victim must be removed from an automobile or from water:

1. Immobilize the back and neck with a reasonably short, wide board. The board should reach down to the victim's buttocks.
2. Place the board behind the victim's head, neck, and back, keeping these body parts in alignment.
3. Tie the victim to the board at the forehead, under the armpits, and around the lower abdomen.
4. *Do not* let the victim's body bend or twist. Move the victim very gently and slowly.

If the victim is not breathing:
Tilt his or her head back slightly to maintain an open airway. Do not twist or rotate the head.

INJURIES AND ILLNESSES

201

If the victim is facedown:
- Get adequate help so that every part of the body can be turned over together in the same position in which it was found.
- Restore breathing if necessary. (See pp. 33–34.)

If the victim must be taken to the hospital by someone other than trained medical personnel:
- If you are unsure whether the injury is to the neck or the back, treat it as if it were a neck injury. (See above.)

See Also: Broken Bones, p. 107; Ear Problems, p. 164; Eye Problems, p. 170; Seizures, p. 237; Tooth Problems, p. 257; Unconsciousness, p. 259.

Headaches are a very common complaint. Most headaches are caused by emotional tension. Other causes include viral infections, sinus infections, allergies, high blood pressure, stroke, brain tumor, meningitis, and head injuries. Mild headaches can usually be relieved by taking aspirin or a nonsteroidal anti-inflammatory medication (such as acetaminophen, ibuprofen, or naproxen) and rest. Applying heat to the back of the neck and sitting or lying down in a dark room or massaging the neck muscles and the scalp may also help relieve headache pain. Any severe or persistent headache requires medical attention.

HEADACHES DURING PREGNANCY

Severe or persistent headaches in the last 3 months of pregnancy can be a sign of danger to both the mother and the baby. Headaches may indicate a serious condition known as toxemia in which the mother's body reacts negatively to the presence of the fetus. Other symptoms of toxemia include swelling of the face and fingers, blurred vision, and rapid weight gain. Any severe or persistent headache at any time during pregnancy requires prompt medical attention.

See Also: Cold-Related Problems, p. 139; Drug Abuse, p. 156; Head, Neck, and Back Injuries, p. 194; Heat-Related Problems, p. 206; Poisoning, p. 225; Stroke, p. 250.

INJURIES AND ILLNESSES

HEART ATTACK

A heart attack is a life-threatening emergency. A heart attack occurs when there is not enough blood and oxygen reaching a portion of the heart due to a narrowing or obstruction of the coronary arteries that supply the heart muscle. A prolonged lack of blood and oxygen can cause part of the heart muscle to die or trigger an abnormal heartbeat that can be fatal. The sooner a victim of a heart attack receives medical treatment, the less damage the heart is likely to undergo and the better the prognosis.

SYMPTOMS

A heart attack can cause any or all of the following symptoms:

- Central chest pain or chest tightness that is severe, crushing (not sharp), constant, and lasts for several minutes (pain may feel like indigestion)
- Chest discomfort that moves through the chest to either arm or the shoulder, neck, jaw, mid-back, or stomach
- Profuse sweating
- Nausea and vomiting
- Extreme weakness
- Anxiety and fearfulness
- Pale skin; blue fingernails and lips
- Extreme shortness of breath
- Dizziness or fainting

WHAT TO DO

If the victim is unconscious and not breathing or is having difficulty breathing:
Call 911 (or your local emergency number). Maintain an open airway. Restore breathing and circulation. (See pp. 31–50.)

If the victim is conscious at the onset of the heart attack:
1. Call 911 (or your local emergency number) and inform medics of a possible heart attack and of the need for oxygen. If this is not possible, take the victim immediately to the nearest hospital emergency department.
2. Gently help the victim to a comfortable position, either sitting up or in a semi-sitting position. A pillow or two may provide greater comfort. The victim should not lie down flat, as this position makes breathing more difficult.
3. If aspirin is available (preferably in chewable form) and the victim is not allergic to it, have him or her take one tablet. Aspirin helps prevent the formation of blood clots.
4. Loosen tight clothing, particularly around the victim's neck.
5. Keep the victim comfortably warm by covering him or her with a blanket or coat.
6. Calm and reassure the victim.

If you are alone and think you're having a heart attack:
1. Call 911 (or your local emergency number) immediately and inform the medics of a possible heart attack and of the need for oxygen.
2. If aspirin is available (preferably in chewable form) and you are not allergic to it, take one tablet. Aspirin helps prevent the formation of blood clots.
3. Get into a comfortable position, either sitting up or in a semi-sitting position. A pillow or two may provide greater comfort.
4. Loosen tight clothing, particularly around your neck.
5. Keep yourself comfortably warm.
6. Do not eat or drink anything.

N O T E : Not all chest pains are symptoms of a heart attack but it is always a good idea to report any chest pains to a doctor.

See Also: Shock, p. 240; Unconsciousness, p. 259.

INJURIES AND ILLNESSES

HEAT CRAMPS

Heat cramps are muscle pains and spasms caused by a loss of salt from the body due to profuse sweating. Strenuous physical activity in hot temperatures can lead to heat cramps. Drinking large amounts of plain water while sweating profusely (without replacing the lost salt) can also contribute to heat cramps. Usually the muscles of the stomach and legs (calves) are affected first. Heat cramps may also be a symptom of heat exhaustion.

SYMPTOMS

Heat cramps may involve any or all of the following symptoms:

- Painful muscle cramping and spasms
- Heavy sweating
- Seizures

WHAT TO DO

1. Have the victim sit quietly in a cool place.
2. If the victim is not vomiting, give a sports drink (check the label to make sure the carbohydrate content does not exceed 6 percent), clear juice, or cool salt water (¼ to ½ teaspoon of table salt or two to four ten-grain salt tablets dissolved in 4 cups of water). Do not give undissolved salt tablets. Give the victim half a glass of liquid every 15 minutes for 1 hour. Stop giving fluids if vomiting occurs.
3. Medical attention is needed because of possible complications.

HEAT EXHAUSTION

Heat exhaustion can occur after prolonged (about 3 to 5 days) exposure to high temperatures and high humidity.

SYMPTOMS

Heat exhaustion can cause any or all of the following symptoms:

- Slightly above normal body temperature
- Pale and clammy skin
- Heavy sweating
- Tiredness or weakness
- Dizziness
- Headache
- Nausea
- Muscle cramps
- Vomiting
- Fainting
- Fast heart rate

WHAT TO DO

1. Move the victim into the shade or to a cooler area.
2. Have the victim lie down.
3. Raise the victim's feet 8 to 12 inches.
4. Loosen the victim's clothing.
5. If the victim is not vomiting, give a sports drink (check the label to make sure the carbohydrate content does not exceed 6 percent), clear juice, or cool salt water (¼ to ½ teaspoon of table salt or two to four ten-grain salt tablets dissolved in 4 cups of water). Do not give undissolved salt tablets.
6. Place cool, wet cloths on the victim's forehead and body.
7. Use a fan to cool the victim while spraying him or her with water from a spray bottle, or place ice bags on the victim's neck, armpits, and groin. If possible, remove the victim to an air-conditioned room.
8. If symptoms are severe, become worse, or last longer than an hour, seek medical attention promptly.

HEATSTROKE (SUNSTROKE)

Heatstroke is a life-threatening emergency. It is a disturbance in the body's heat-regulating system caused by an extremely high body temperature resulting from exposure to heat and an inability of the body to cool itself.

SYMPTOMS

Heatstroke can cause any or all of the following symptoms:

- Extremely high body temperature (often 106°F or higher)
- Rapid and strong pulse

- Unconsciousness or confusion
- Fast breathing
- Vomiting and diarrhea
- Seizures
- Incoordination

WHAT TO DO

If body temperature reaches 105°F:

1. Undress the victim and put him or her into a tub of cold water if possible. Otherwise, spray the victim with a hose, sponge bare skin with cool water or rubbing alcohol, or apply cold packs to the victim's neck, armpits, and groin.
2. Continue treatment until body temperature is lowered to 101°F or 102°F.
3. Do not overchill; check the victim's temperature constantly. If body temperature rises again, repeat the cooling process.
4. *Do not* give the victim aspirin, acetaminophen, or other pain relievers; alcoholic beverages; or stimulants (such as coffee or tea).
5. Dry off the victim once temperature is lowered. Place the victim in front of a fan or an air conditioner.
6. Seek medical attention promptly, preferably at the nearest hospital emergency department.

Preventing Heat-Related Problems

Infants, older people, and those who are overweight or have an endocrine disease (such as diabetes) or a skin disease (such as psoriasis) are most susceptible to heat-related problems. Here are some steps you can take to avoid problems from overexposure to heat:

- Until your body is accustomed to hot weather (about a week for adults and 2 weeks for children), limit outdoor activities to 90 minutes a day. It's best to exercise before 8 AM or after 6 PM.
- Wear loose, lightweight clothing.
- Drink 8 ounces of fluid 15 minutes before engaging in a vigorous outdoor activity and drink 8 to 12 ounces of fluid every 30 minutes during the activity.
- Avoid alcohol, amphetamines, or antihistamines when exercising in hot weather.

HYPERVENTILATION

Hyperventilation is breathing faster and more deeply than normal due to tension or emotional upset. The person feels as if he or she is not getting enough air into the lungs. Feeling out of breath, he or she increases breathing in an attempt to take in more air. As rapid breathing continues, the level of carbon dioxide in the blood is lowered, causing muscle tightness in the throat and chest, which further aggravates the symptoms.

SYMPTOMS

Hyperventilation can cause any or all of the following symptoms:

- Light-headedness
- Numbness and tingling in the hands and feet and around the mouth and lips
- Feeling of tightness in the throat
- Muscle twitching
- Difficulty getting a deep, "satisfying" breath
- Convulsions

WHAT TO DO

1. Encourage the person to relax and try to breathe slowly and easily.
2. If breathing does not return to normal, seek medical attention. Even after breathing returns to normal, it is a good idea to see a doctor to determine the underlying cause of the hyperventilation.

See Also: Seizures, p. 237.

LEAD POISONING

Lead poisoning is a disease that results from an excessive level of lead in the body. Lead poisoning most often occurs in young children who nibble on paint chips, plaster, putty, and other substances containing lead. Brain damage may result from prolonged exposure to lead. It is extremely important to seek medical attention as soon as lead poisoning is suspected.

SYMPTOMS

Lead poisoning can cause any or all of the following symptoms:

- Vomiting
- Weakness
- Fatigue
- Irritability
- Trouble sleeping
- Fever
- Paleness
- Convulsions
- Abdominal pain
- Poor appetite

WHAT TO DO

For any symptoms of lead poisoning, or to examine the possibility of lead poisoning in the absence of symptoms, see a doctor for a complete examination and evaluation, which will include testing the level of lead in the blood.

Preventing Lead Poisoning

Here are some steps you can take to help keep your children safe from lead poisoning:

- Have your children wash their hands and face after playing outside and before eating.
- Wash toys often; discard any toys that might have lead-based paint (such as those made in other countries).

- Give your child foods high in iron and calcium (both of which help prevent lead absorption by the body) and low in fat (fat promotes lead absorption); don't store food in opened cans or in pottery.
- Use cold tap water for cooking (hot water draws lead from pipes). Before using cold water from the tap, let it run for a few minutes.
- Remove chipping and peeling paint and paint dust. Leave the house during remodeling.

See Also: Rashes, p. 233; Seizures, p. 237; Unconsciousness, p. 259; Vomiting, p. 262.

INJURIES AND ILLNESSES

LICE INFESTATION

Lice are small (about ⅛ inch), wingless insects that can infest any part of the body, but are usually found on children's heads. They are very contagious and spread easily among children in school. Female lice lay a daily batch of tiny, white eggs (nits) that attach firmly to the sides of hairs, usually close to the scalp.

SYMPTOMS

A lice infestation can cause any or all of the following symptoms:

- Intense itching at the site of infestation
- Redness of the skin
- Enlarged lymph nodes in the neck

WHAT TO DO

If you know for sure it is a lice infestation on the scalp:
1. Use shampoo with the active ingredient permethrin (check the label); carefully follow the instructions on the container.
2. After shampooing, comb through the hair using a special fine-toothed comb to remove any nits. Use the comb frequently to check for the presence of lice or eggs and to determine if the treatment has worked.
3. Spray any furniture and bedding that have been used in the previous 3 days with permethrin.
4. Dry-clean or machine wash at the hottest setting all exposed towels, sheets, and clothing. Iron them if possible.
5. Place small, potentially contaminated objects in plastic bags for 2 weeks, or until the lice are no longer visible.
6. Throw out all exposed combs and brushes.
7. If your child is infested, report it immediately to his or her school.

8. If the lice reappear within a week after using the shampoo, see a physician.

If the infestation is in another area of the body, such as the genitals:

1. See a physician; he or she may recommend a special shampoo or lotion.
2. Inform your sexual partner and anyone with whom you have had close physical contact so that they can also seek treatment.

See Also: Scabies Infestation, p. 236.

LIGHTNING STRIKE

Being struck by lightning is a serious incident. Electricity generated by lightning disrupts the electrical activity in the brain that controls breathing and heartbeat and can make the victim's heart stop beating. Heat generated by the lightning can cause severe burns and internal injuries. Broken bones can occur from sudden, strenuous muscle contractions. The victim may also be injured if he or she is thrown into the air from the force of the lightning strike. You can immediately touch a person who has been struck by lightning because the source of the electrical power is no longer present. Most lightning injuries occur between noon and 6 PM.

SYMPTOMS

A lightning strike can cause any or all of the following symptoms:

- Disorientation, confusion, or dizziness
- Inability to speak
- Unconsciousness or seizures
- Absence of breathing
- Burn marks
- Bleeding
- Temporary blindness
- Ruptured eardrum
- Amnesia that lasts for hours or even days
- Internal or external injuries

WHAT TO DO

1. Call 911 (or your local emergency number). Maintain an open airway. Restore breathing and circulation if necessary. (See pp. 31–50.)

2. While waiting for medical help to arrive, provide first aid for any problems such as bleeding (see p. 96) or broken bones (see p. 107).
3. Calm and reassure the victim.

Preventing Lightning Injuries

Here are some steps you can take to avoid a lightning injury:

• Be aware of violent, fast-moving storms in your area. Lightning can strike before a storm is overhead.
• Seek shelter in a large, substantial building; shelters such as tents or sheds offer little protection.
• Remain in an all-metal vehicle; a cloth-top convertible offers less protection.
• Outdoors, stay away from metal objects such as power lines, ski lifts, and fences. Do not open your umbrella if you can hear thunder or see lightning.
• Do not stand near tall trees. If you are in a wooded area, seek shelter in a thick growth of young trees or saplings.
• If you are in an open area, seek shelter in a dry cave or ditch (make sure there is no water around it). Crouch there rolled up like a ball.
• If you are swimming or boating, get to shore as quickly as possible or stay underneath a bridge.
• If you are indoors, try not to use the telephone or computer modem. Stay away from fireplaces and open doors and windows.

INJURIES AND ILLNESSES

LUMPS AND BUMPS

Lumps and bumps are common injuries. Any bump on the head resulting from an injury may be serious and requires medical attention.

WHAT TO DO

- As soon as the injury occurs, apply cold compresses or an ice pack to the affected area to decrease swelling and alleviate pain.
- Seek medical attention promptly for a lump on the head if a person has bleeding from the ears, nose, or mouth; unconsciousness; a change in pulse; severe headache; difficulty breathing; convulsions; severe vomiting; pupils of unequal size; slurred speech; a generally poor appearance; or a personality change.
- If a bump is a result of a head injury, check that the person is not unconscious by awakening him or her every ½ hour for the first 2 hours, every 2 hours for the next 24 hours, every 4 hours for the second 24 hours, and every 8 hours for the third 24 hours.
- Seek medical attention for any severe lump or bump on any part of the body.

See Also: Broken Bones, p. 107; Bruises, p. 119; Eye Problems, p. 170; Head, Neck, and Back Injuries, p. 194; Headaches, p. 203; Unconsciousness, p. 259.

MERCURY POISONING

Mercury, the silver-colored liquid metal in fever thermometers, is a poisonous substance that can be absorbed by the body. Other sources of metallic mercury include thermostats and blood pressure monitors. The most dangerous way to be exposed to this form of mercury is by inhaling it over a long period of time, usually in an industrial workplace. Swallowing small amounts of metallic mercury, such as that in a fever thermometer, is usually not harmful. Without treatment, severe mercury poisoning can cause birth defects, damage organs, or even be fatal. Students sometimes steal mercury from school chemistry labs to play with it at home or conduct their own experiments. If you notice a substance resembling mercury in a glass jar, immediately call your local environmental health department, board of health, poison control center, or doctor to find out how to dispose of the metal properly.

SYMPTOMS

Contact with mercury or mercury poisoning can cause any or all of the following symptoms:

- An allergic-type rash on the skin (on skin contact)
- Nausea, vomiting, diarrhea, and abdominal pain (on inhalation)
- Shortness of breath or coughing (on inhalation)

WHAT TO DO

If the amount of mercury is greater than that from a small fever thermometer or if mercury from a thermometer spills on a porous surface (such as upholstered furniture or unfinished wood):

1. Do not touch the mercury or try to clean it up, even with a vacuum cleaner.

2. Call your local environmental health department, board of health, poison control center, or doctor (even if no one has any noticeable symptoms).
3. Open the windows to ventilate the area.
4. Leave the area until a health professional has evaluated the situation and the mercury has been cleaned up.

If the amount of mercury is small (such as that in a fever thermometer) and it spills on a nonporous surface (such as ceramic tile or finished wood):
1. Remove any gold jewelry you are wearing (mercury adheres to gold) and be careful to avoid any skin contact with the mercury (only special gloves designed to handle hazardous materials are protective against mercury poisoning).
2. Use an index card or stiff paper to scoop up the mercury droplets and place them in a glass jar with a tight lid or in a reclosable plastic bag. Alternatively, you can use masking tape, duct tape, or cellophane tape to remove the mercury; put the wad of tape and mercury in a glass jar or reclosable plastic bag.
3. Call your local environmental health department, board of health, poison control center, or doctor and ask how to dispose of the mercury.
4. Ventilate the area of the spill for at least 2 days.

MISCARRIAGE

A miscarriage is the loss of a fetus before the 12th week of pregnancy. Miscarriages are common and occur in approximately 10 percent of pregnancies, usually in the first 3 months.

The first signs of a possible miscarriage are usually bleeding followed by lower abdominal cramping. Although vaginal bleeding and/or cramping do not always indicate a miscarriage, if either of these symptoms appears, notify a doctor immediately. If heavy or continuous bleeding occurs, seek medical attention immediately, preferably at the nearest hospital emergency department.

Until the doctor is notified and can give specific instructions, the woman should rest in bed. If any material such as tissue or unusual-looking clots passes from the vagina, save it (preferably in a container in the refrigerator) and bring it to the doctor's office for inspection.

See Also: Abdominal Pain, p. 59; Childbirth, Emergency, p. 130; Pregnancy Danger Signs, p. 228.

INJURIES AND ILLNESSES

Pain in the muscles is common and usually not serious. Muscle pain is often caused by tension, infection, fatigue (particularly in children), and overexercising. Gently massaging the area, taking a warm bath, applying warm, wet compresses, and resting are often helpful in relieving the pain. Stretching exercises (begun slowly) also may be helpful. Any pain that is severe or prolonged needs medical attention.

Muscle cramps can be particularly painful and often occur in the middle of the night, usually in the feet, calves, or thighs. Cramps usually result from fatigue or from keeping a limb in one position for a prolonged period. Massaging the area to relax the muscle is usually effective, because it stimulates local circulation, but do not massage the muscle if the problem could be heat cramps (see p. 206).

If the cramp is in the foot, turn the toes up toward your body. If the cramp is in the calf, stand up (with most of your weight on the unaffected leg) and massage the cramp. For a cramp in the thigh, lie down while massaging the area. Applying a heating pad or taking a warm bath can also be helpful.

Cramps in the legs and thighs often occur during pregnancy. The treatment is the same as described above. Also, be sure to get plenty of rest.

See Also: Bites and Stings, p. 72; Broken Bones, p. 107; Bruises, p. 119; Cold-Related Problems, p. 139; Dislocations, p. 151; Food Poisoning, p. 185; Heat-Related Problems, p. 206; Muscle Strains, p. 221; Sprains, p. 248; and Sports First Aid, p. 271–336.

MUSCLE STRAINS

A strain results from pulling or overexerting a muscle. Back strains are common injuries.

SYMPTOMS

Muscle strains can cause one or both of the following symptoms:

• A dull pain in the affected muscle that worsens with movement
• Swelling

WHAT TO DO

1. Rest the affected area immediately.
2. Apply ice or a cold compress to the area intermittently (30 minutes on, 30 minutes off) to decrease swelling during the first 24 hours after the injury.
3. After 24 hours, apply warm, wet compresses to the area.
4. If possible, elevate the strained area above the level of the heart.
5. Seek medical attention if the pain or swelling is severe.

See Also: Muscle Aches and Pains, p. 220; Sports First Aid, pp. 271–336.

A nosebleed can be caused by a blow to the nose, scratching the nose, repeated nose blowing that irritates the mucous membrane, dry air, or an infection. Most nosebleeds that occur in children are not serious and usually stop within a few minutes. Those that occur in the elderly, however, may be serious and may require treatment at a hospital emergency department. Recurring nosebleeds may indicate an underlying medical problem and should be evaluated by a doctor.

WHAT TO DO

1. Have the victim sit down and lean forward, keeping the mouth open so that blood or clots will not obstruct the airway.
2. Squeeze the sides of the nose together for approximately 10 minutes. (Squeeze the nose below the bone, not on the top of the nose.)
3. Release slowly. *Do not* allow the victim to blow or touch the nose.
4. If bleeding continues, squeeze the nose closed again for 5 minutes. Be sure that the victim is not swallowing blood.
5. Place a cold cloth or ice in a cloth over the bridge of the victim's nose and face to help constrict blood vessels.
6. Seek medical attention if bleeding continues, an injury is involved, you suspect a broken nose, the victim complains of dizziness or light-headedness, or the victim is pale or has a fast heart rate.
7. *Do not* let the victim irritate or blow the nose for several hours after bleeding stops.

PLANT IRRITATIONS

Poison ivy, poison oak, and poison sumac are three plants that can cause a reaction on the skin of sensitive people. An oily substance on the plants causes the irritation. You can be exposed to the plant toxins indirectly by touching pets that have had contact with the plants. Burning the leaves of the plants can cause breathing problems in sensitive people.

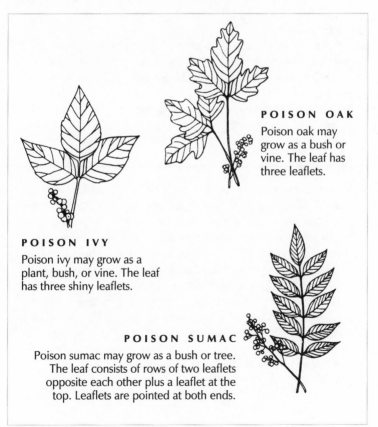

POISON OAK

Poison oak may grow as a bush or vine. The leaf has three leaflets.

POISON IVY

Poison ivy may grow as a plant, bush, or vine. The leaf has three shiny leaflets.

POISON SUMAC

Poison sumac may grow as a bush or tree. The leaf consists of rows of two leaflets opposite each other plus a leaflet at the top. Leaflets are pointed at both ends.

SYMPTOMS

Contact with poison ivy, poison oak, and poison sumac can cause any or all of the following symptoms:

- Redness of the skin
- Blisters
- Itching
- Headache
- Fever

WHAT TO DO

1. Wear gloves if you are helping someone who has been exposed to any of these plants. As soon as possible, remove clothes and thoroughly wash the affected area with soap and water.
2. Sponge the affected area with rubbing alcohol.
3. Apply calamine lotion to help relieve itching. A colloid oatmeal bath (available in most drugstores) can also help relieve itching.
4. Seek medical attention if the symptoms are severe or don't improve in 2 to 3 days.

Preventing Reactions to Plants

If you know you are allergic to poison ivy, poison oak, or poison sumac, or you know you will be in an area where you might come in contact with the plants, ask your doctor about using a protective lotion containing the active ingredient bentoquatum to block a reaction. The over-the-counter lotion is available in drugstores. Apply the lotion to exposed skin 15 minutes before possible contact with the plants and every 4 hours thereafter for continued protection. To be extra safe, you should also wear protective clothing to avoid exposure to the plants. You can remove the lotion from your skin later with soap and water. *Do not* use bentoquatum if you have already developed a rash.

It is extremely important to call the poison control center, hospital emergency department, a doctor, or 911 (or your local emergency number) for instructions before doing anything for a person who has swallowed a poison. When calling, be sure to give the following information:

- Victim's age
- Name of the poison
- How much poison was swallowed
- When poison was swallowed
- Whether or not the victim has vomited
- How much time it will take to get the victim to a medical facility

Emergency treatment for victims of swallowed poisons consists of:

- Seeking prompt medical attention.
- Diluting the poison with water or milk as quickly as possible. *Do not* give fruit juice or vinegar to neutralize the poison.
- Getting the poison out of the victim. Inducing vomiting is rarely done, and should be undertaken on medical advice only (preferably from the staff at the poison control center).

Do not induce vomiting if the victim is unconscious or is having seizures. *Do not* induce vomiting if you do not know what the victim has swallowed.

Do not induce vomiting if the victim has swallowed:
- A strong acid or alkali such as toilet bowl cleaner, rust remover, chlorine bleach, dishwasher detergent, or glucose-test tablets
- A petroleum product such as kerosene, gasoline, furniture polish, charcoal lighter fluid, or paint thinner

INJURIES AND ILLNESSES

If vomited, strong acids and alkalis may cause further damage to the throat and esophagus. Petroleum products, if vomited, can be drawn into the lungs and cause chemical pneumonia. It is important to note, however, that the poison control center may recommend inducing vomiting for some of the products mentioned above (particularly the petroleum products) because of other chemicals in the swallowed product that may be even more harmful to the body.

Always follow the instructions of the poison control center. If the victim vomits, whether induced or spontaneously, keep the victim facedown with the head lower than the rest of the body so that he or she will not choke on the vomit. Place a small child facedown across your knees. Be sure to take the poison container and any vomited material to the hospital for inspection.

N O T E : The information or instructions on labels of poisonous substances are not always correct, particularly if the container is old. It is always best to consult the poison control center if possible.

WHAT TO DO

If the victim is not breathing:
1. Call the poison control center, 911 (or your local emergency number), an ambulance, the fire department, or other rescue personnel for transportation to the hospital.
2. Maintain an open airway. Restore breathing and circulation if necessary. (See pp. 31–50.)
3. Take the poison container and any vomited material to the hospital with the victim.

If the victim is unconscious or having seizures:
1. Seek medical attention immediately. Call 911 (or your local emergency number), the poison control center, an ambulance, the fire department, or other rescue personnel for transportation to the hospital. The victim should be transported lying on his or her side or stomach.
2. Maintain an open airway if possible. Restore breathing and circulation if necessary. (See pp. 31–50.)
3. Loosen tight clothing around the victim's neck and waist. *Do not* give any fluids to the victim. *Do not* try to induce vomiting.

If the victim vomits on his or her own, turn his or her head to the side so that he or she will not choke on the vomit.

4. Take the poison container and any vomited material to the hospital with the victim.

If the victim is conscious:

1. Have someone else (if possible) call 911 (or your local emergency number), the poison control center, hospital emergency department, or a doctor for instructions while you continue to care for the victim.

2. Induce vomiting *only* if told to do so by medical personnel. Induce vomiting only if the swallowed poison is *not* an acid, alkali, or petroleum product. Vomiting may be induced by giving an adult or child over 12 years old (unless of low weight) 2 tablespoons of syrup of ipecac; a child between the ages of 1 and 11 years, 1 tablespoon; and an infant under 1 year, 2 teaspoons. Follow with one or two glasses of water or milk. If vomiting does not occur within 15 to 20 minutes, repeat dosage of ipecac only once. *Do not* give mustard or table salt to the victim to induce vomiting.

If syrup of ipecac is not available, the poison control center may recommend giving the victim activated charcoal if you have it; carefully follow the directions the center gives you. (Activated charcoal, which is available at drugstores, blocks the stomach's absorption of the poison.)

If vomiting does not occur:

3. Seek medical attention immediately. Take the poison container to the hospital with the victim.

If vomiting occurs:

3. Keep the victim facedown with the head lower than the rest of the body or lying on his or her left side to prevent choking on vomit. Place a small child facedown across your knees. Seek medical attention immediately. Take the poison container and any vomited material to the hospital with the victim.

See Also: Burns (Chemical Burns), p. 126; Carbon Monoxide Poisoning, p. 128; Diarrhea, p. 148; Drug Abuse, p. 156; Food Poisoning, p. 185; Lead Poisoning, p. 210; Mercury Poisoning, p. 217; Rashes, p. 233; Seizures, p. 237; Unconsciousness, p. 259.

INJURIES AND ILLNESSES

PREGNANCY DANGER SIGNS

Certain symptoms during pregnancy should be reported immediately to a doctor. They may or may not indicate a serious condition, but only a doctor can evaluate the situation. The symptoms to report immediately include:

- *Any* vaginal bleeding
- Stomach pain or cramps
- Persistent vomiting
- Severe, persistent headaches
- Swelling of the face or fingers
- Blurring or dimness of vision
- Chills and fever
- Sudden leaking of water from the vagina
- Convulsions
- Difficulty breathing

See Also: Childbirth, Emergency, p. 130; Miscarriage, p. 219.

RAPE/SEXUAL ASSAULT

Sexual assault is forced or manipulated sexual contact without consent or agreement. Sexual assault includes forced vaginal or anal intercourse, oral sex, or penetration with an object. These activities are usually referred to as rape. Sexual assault also includes involuntary sexual contact such as forced touching or fondling.

Rape is a crime in every state. Some state laws have been expanded to include rape in marriage and between individuals of the same sex. The motives of the rapist are dominance and control.

If you are alone and you have been raped, or if another person has been raped, call the police immediately to report the crime. Next, call a relative, friend, or rape hotline (or other community agency with rape counseling available). Then call your doctor or the hospital emergency department to let them know that a rape has occurred and that you or another individual will be seeking medical treatment.

SYMPTOMS

Injuries from a sexual assault vary according to the manner of attack and may involve any or all of the following symptoms:

- Blood on underwear
- Bleeding from the vagina or anus
- Cuts, burns, bruises (especially on inner thighs or in genital area)
- Fearfulness, anxiety, depression, shame, embarrassment

WHAT TO DO

- Treat noticeable injuries, such as cuts, bruises, or burns.
- Do not allow the victim to take a shower, bathe, brush his or her teeth, or eat or drink anything.

229

- Comfort the victim and provide emotional support; be nonjudgmental.
- Believe the victim.
- Do not leave the victim alone.
- Take the victim to a hospital emergency department or doctor's office immediately for further treatment.

IF A RAPE HAS OCCURRED, DO NOT ALLOW THE VICTIM TO:

Change clothes.   Take a shower.   Brush his or her teeth.   Eat or drink.

BE SURE TO:

Call the police.   Call a relative or friend to assist you.   Call a doctor, a hospital emergency department, or an abuse hotline.

The rape victim will probably be given a private room or taken to a private area at the physician's office or hospital emergency department. A social worker, police officer, and medical personnel may all be present to help. The victim may be asked several times to describe what happened and to give a description of the assailant.

A physician will recommend that the victim have a complete physical examination. The exam is performed with the victim's consent to protect him or her from disease and to collect physical evidence of the assault. The exam will include taking samples from the mouth, vagina, and rectum, and testing for sexually transmitted infections such as chlamydia, gonorrhea, syphilis, and HIV. A test may also be done for a pre-existing pregnancy. The tests will determine the victim's health status at the time the crime occurred.

The victim will be asked to seek follow-up medical treatment, depending on the injuries and test results. He or she should also seek counseling for assistance in handling the emotional aspects of the assault.

DATE RAPE DRUGS

Date rape drugs are powerful tranquilizers that alter consciousness and can induce the sleepiness of a deep coma within 30 minutes. They get their name from the most common situation in which they are used: a prospective sexual assailant, usually a man, targets a potential rape victim, usually a woman, and secretly places a pill or a small amount of a colorless, odorless, tasteless liquid into the woman's alcoholic beverage at a party or bar. The drugs that are used most frequently for this purpose include flunitrazepam (known on the street as the forget-me pill, R-2, or roach) and gamma hydroxyl butyrate (known on the street as scoop, liquid G, or grievous bodily harm). Alcohol intensifies the action of these drugs.

SYMPTOMS

A person who has been given a date rape drug will have any or all of the following symptoms, which can last up to 8 hours:

- Drowsiness within half an hour of drinking a beverage or ingesting a pill containing the tranquilizer
- Complete or partial amnesia; the victim may later recall only snapshot-like images of the sexual assault
- Incoordination
- Slow breathing
- Unexplained bruises
- Confused behavior
- Impaired judgment

INJURIES AND ILLNESSES

WHAT TO DO

1. Call 911 (or your local emergency number) or take the person to the nearest hospital emergency department. Doctors can perform examinations and tests that can help determine what happened; these procedures are most reliable when they are performed soon after an assault.
2. Treat any injuries.
3. Tell the victim not to bathe or shower, eat or drink, change clothes, or brush his or her teeth.
4. Give the victim emotional support.

Avoiding Date Rape Drugs

Here are some steps you can take to avoid being the victim of a drug-induced date rape:

- Closely watch the preparation of your drinks.
- Do not set your glass down or look away from it; keep your hand over the top of your drink if you have to look away or are distracted for a moment.
- Do not drink any liquid that has a white film on the surface or on the glass (this can indicate a partially dissolved drug).
- Be careful when getting drinks from punch bowls or large containers of alcoholic beverages when you are at a party at which you don't know or trust the host or other guests (large containers of beverages are easy to contaminate intentionally).

Skin rashes occur for many reasons including allergic reactions, fever, heat, or infectious diseases. Some rashes may indicate a serious problem. Medical attention should always be sought if blue, purple, or blood-red spots appear (these may mean bleeding in and under the skin); the rash becomes worse; signs of infection such as pus or red streaks occur; itching is severe; or if other symptoms are present.

BITES AND STINGS

Rashes may appear after insect stings, tick bites, brown recluse spider bites, and rat bites. Rashes that result from bites and stings should be seen by a doctor. Some may rapidly lead to breathing difficulties. (See Bites and Stings, p. 72.)

INFECTIONS

Rashes are present with many infectious diseases. Infections that can cause rashes include chickenpox, measles, rubella, Lyme disease, Rocky Mountain spotted fever, scarlet fever, certain forms of meningitis, roseola infantum, and infectious mononucleosis.

REACTION TO MEDICATIONS

A skin reaction may appear with any medication, although these rashes are more likely to appear with the use of powerful drugs such as barbiturates, tranquilizers, and antibiotics. If a rash appears while the person is on a medication, call the doctor immediately to see if a rash is to be expected from the illness for which the medication was prescribed, or if it is a reaction to the drug.

INJURIES AND ILLNESSES

HEAT RASH

Heat rash, or prickly heat, is a common rash caused by high body temperature due to fever or hot, humid weather. The sweat ducts are blocked and the area affected is covered with tiny red pinpoints. Both prevention and treatment consist of avoiding extreme heat.

Dusting powders and soothing lotions are also helpful. Light, dry, loose clothing should be worn in hot weather. Heat rash usually disappears in a cool environment. If heat rash persists, a doctor should be consulted.

HIVES

Hives is an allergic reaction to various substances characterized by large or small, irregularly shaped and sized, bumpy swellings that cause stinging, burning, and itching. Animal hairs, feathers, laundry detergents, plants, fabrics, dyes, medications, and viral infections may cause hives. Food is a common offender, particularly chocolate, nuts, berries, and seafood. For first attacks of hives, it is best to seek medical attention. If hives has occurred before, follow previous instructions of the doctor. If hives persists, see your doctor. If other symptoms are present, such as difficulty breathing or swallowing, seek medical attention promptly; this could be a severe, life-threatening allergic reaction called anaphylactic shock (see p. 240).

PLANT REACTIONS

Contact with plants often produces a rash in sensitive persons. The most common offenders are poison ivy, poison oak, and poison sumac. (See Plant Irritations, p. 223.)

RASHES IN INFANTS

Infants often have rashes. The most common is diaper rash, which is not dangerous but can cause a lot of discomfort. Diaper rash usually is a burn that occurs when bacteria react with urine on the skin and break down the urine into ammonia. Diaper rash may also be caused by fungi from an infant's stool. Thorough skin cleansing followed by drying will help. Very absorbent, dry diapers should be used and changed frequently. Various ointments are available, but it is best to ask a doctor for specific instructions.

A common rash in newborns appears during the early weeks of life. It may appear anywhere on the body and often moves from one place to another. The affected area should be kept clean and dry. It is always a good idea to report all infant rashes to a doctor.

Rashes on infants can also be caused by food allergies and by contact with substances such as clothes washed in strong detergents, rubber in pants, skin-care products, and soap left behind the ears. These rashes should also be reported to a doctor.

INJURIES AND ILLNESSES

SCABIES INFESTATION

Scabies is an infestation by a mite that burrows into the skin. Scabies infestations are very contagious—spreading from person to person and from furniture, clothing, or pets. Common sites of infestation include areas between the fingers and toes, the inside of the elbow or wrist, under the armpits, or on the genitals.

SYMPTOMS

A scabies infestation can cause any or all of the following symptoms, which usually develop about 3 to 4 weeks after the initial contact:

- Intense itching that is usually worse at night and after bathing
- Red, raised sores on the skin

WHAT TO DO

1. See a physician; he or she may recommend a special body shampoo to eliminate the mites.
2. Spray your furniture with gamma benzene hexachloride spray. *Do not* spray your skin with this product.
3. Wash all contaminated clothing, bedding, and towels in very hot water the morning after you begin treatment. Iron everything, if possible, to help kill the mites.

A seizure (convulsion) results from a disturbance in the electrical activity of the brain, causing a series of uncontrollable muscle movements. These may occur during a state of total or partial unconsciousness and there may be a temporary loss of breathing. Most seizures last 1 to 2 minutes.

Seizures may occur with a head injury, brain tumor, poisoning, electric shock, withdrawal from drugs, heatstroke, scorpion bites, poisonous snakebites, hyperventilation, or high fever. Seizures also occur in people who have epilepsy, a disorder that results when brain cells temporarily become overactive and release too much electrical energy. A person with epilepsy sometimes has a warning sensation (aura)—a particular taste, smell, or hallucination—that indicates a seizure is about to occur.

You should consider a seizure a medical emergency unless the person having it is known to have epilepsy. However, a person with epilepsy requires emergency medical attention if he or she has a seizure that lasts longer than 5 minutes.

A person having a seizure is not in danger of biting off or swallowing his or her tongue. *Do not* put any object into the victim's mouth. Injuries may result from falling during the seizure or from bumping into surrounding objects.

SYMPTOMS

Seizures may involve any or all of the following symptoms:

- A short cry or scream
- Rigid muscles followed by jerky, twitching movements
- Breathing temporarily stops
- Face and lips turn blue
- Eyes roll upward
- Rapid heart rate
- Loss of bladder and bowel control

INJURIES AND ILLNESSES

- Drooling or foaming at the mouth (foam may be bloody)
- Unresponsiveness
- Sleepiness and confusion after the seizure is over

WHAT TO DO

- Call 911 (or your local emergency number) if the person having the seizure is not known to have epilepsy or if a person with epilepsy has a seizure that lasts longer than 5 minutes.
- If the victim starts to fall, try to catch him or her and lay him or her down gently.
- Remove any surrounding objects that the victim might strike during the seizure, or remove the victim from dangerous surroundings (such as stairs, glass doors, or a fireplace).
- If breathing stops and does not start again immediately, maintain an open airway (see pp. 31–50). Check to make sure the victim's tongue is not blocking his or her throat. Restore breathing if necessary after the seizure.
- Make sure that the victim does not injure himself or herself but *do not* interfere with his or her movements. *Do not* try to hold the victim down, as muscle tears or fractures may result.
- *Do not* force any object such as a spoon or pencil between the victim's teeth.
- *Do not* throw any liquid on the victim's face or into his or her mouth.
- Loosen tight clothing around the victim's neck and waist.
- After the seizure is over, turn the victim's head to the side or place the victim on his or her side to prevent choking on secretions, blood, or vomit.
- Keep the victim lying down after the seizure is over, as he or she may be confused for a while.
- If necessary, ask bystanders to leave the area.
- Check for other injuries, such as bleeding and broken bones, and administer appropriate treatment.
- Stay with the victim while he or she recovers.

SEIZURES IN INFANTS AND CHILDREN

Seizures in young children are fairly common. The most frequent cause is a rapid rise in temperature due to an acute infection.

These seizures are called febrile seizures and usually occur in children between 1 and 4 years of age. Febrile seizures seldom last longer than 2 to 3 minutes. Although all seizures in young children must be taken seriously, they are usually more frightening to see than dangerous. The symptoms for febrile seizures are the same as for regular seizures (see pp. 237–238).

WHAT TO DO

1. Do not panic.
2. If breathing stops and does not start again immediately, maintain an open airway (see pp. 31–50). Check to make sure the victim's tongue is not blocking his or her throat. Restore breathing if necessary after the seizure.
3. After the seizure, turn the child's head to one side or place the child on his or her side so that he or she will not choke on vomit.
4. Remove the child's clothes and sponge his or her body with lukewarm water to help reduce the fever. *Do not* use rubbing alcohol and *do not* place the child in a tub of water because he or she may inhale the water during the seizure. *Do not* throw water on the child's face or into his or her mouth.
5. Have someone else call the child's doctor during the seizure so you do not have to leave the child unattended. If this is impossible, call the doctor when the seizure is over. If the doctor is not available, take the child to the nearest hospital emergency department.

See Also: Drug Abuse, p. 156; Fever, p. 180; Head, Neck, and Back Injuries, p. 194; Headaches, p. 203; Heat-Related Problems, p. 206; Poisoning, p. 225; Pregnancy Danger Signs, p. 228; and Shock, p. 240.

INJURIES AND ILLNESSES

Shock is a life-threatening situation in which the body's vital functions, such as breathing and heartbeat, are seriously threatened by insufficient oxygenated blood reaching body tissues, such as the lungs, the brain, and the heart. Shock usually results from a serious illness or injury—such as severe bleeding or burns, a heart attack, spinal injury, persistent vomiting or diarrhea, perforation of an organ, poisoning, a severe allergic reaction, or a bacterial infection in the blood.

ANAPHYLACTIC SHOCK

Anaphylactic shock is a life-threatening condition that results from a severe allergic reaction to an insect sting, medication, or food.

SYMPTOMS

Anaphylactic shock can cause any or all of the following symptoms:

- Weakness
- Coughing and/or wheezing
- Difficulty breathing
- Severe itching or hives
- Stomach cramps
- Nausea and vomiting
- Anxiety
- Bluish tinge to skin
- Dizziness
- Collapse
- Unconsciousness
- Weak pulse

If this is the first time the victim has had a severe allergic reaction:
1. Call 911 (or your local emergency number). Maintain an open airway. Restore breathing and circulation if necessary. (See pp. 31–50.)
2. Keep the victim lying down. Turn the victim's head to the side if he or she is vomiting, or position the victim on his or her side.
3. Keep the victim comfortable.

If the person has had a severe allergic reaction before and he or she has an anaphylaxis emergency kit:
1. Help the person administer the injection of adrenaline. If he or she is unable to give himself or herself the injection, give it by following the directions in the kit.
2. Call 911 (or your local emergency number) or transport the person to the nearest hospital emergency department.
3. Keep the victim lying down unless he or she is short of breath; then let the victim sit up slowly.
4. Keep the victim comfortable and quiet.

SHOCK FROM SEVERE INJURY

Shock can occur with injuries that result in heavy loss of blood or other body fluids or too little oxygen reaching the lungs.

SYMPTOMS

Shock from severe bleeding can cause any or all of the following symptoms:

- Pale or bluish and cool skin
- Moist and clammy skin
- Overall weakness
- Rapid (over 100 beats per minute) and weak pulse
- Increased rate of breathing; shallow and irregular breathing or deep sighing
- Restlessness, anxiety
- Unusual thirst
- Vomiting

- Dull, sunken look to the eyes; widely dilated pupils
- Unresponsiveness
- Blotchy or streaked skin
- Unconsciousness (in severe cases)

WHAT TO DO

1. Call 911 (or your local emergency number). Maintain an open airway. Restore breathing and circulation if necessary. (See pp. 31–50.)
2. Treat the cause of shock, such as breathing difficulties, bleeding, or severe pain.
3. Keep the victim lying down. Position him or her on the side with his or her head extended back slightly (with jaws open) to prevent choking on fluids or vomit. *Do not* move the victim if he or she has head, neck, or back injuries unless the victim is in danger of further injury.
4. Elevate the victim's feet 8 to 12 inches unless he or she is unconscious or has injuries to the neck, spine, head, back, chest, lower face, or jaw. If he or she is having trouble breathing, raise his or her head and shoulders slightly to help keep the airway clear.
5. Check to see that the victim is not getting chilled. Keep him or her comfortably warm. If possible, place a blanket under a victim who is on the ground or on a damp surface.
6. Watch the victim very closely for changes in consciousness. Look for other injuries such as internal bleeding (see p. 100) and broken bones (see p. 107) and give first aid for those problems. This may decrease the severity of the shock. *Do not* give the victim fluids if he or she is unconscious, having seizures, likely to need surgery, has a brain injury, has a stomach wound, is vomiting, or is bleeding from the rectum. Stop fluids if vomiting occurs.
7. Reassure the victim. Gentleness, kindness, and understanding play an important role in treating a victim in shock.
8. If possible, obtain information about the nature of the accident.

INSULIN SHOCK

Insulin shock can occur in individuals who have diabetes when there is too little blood glucose (sugar) in the blood. The condition arises when the person takes too much insulin, or eats too little food after taking insulin or other diabetes medications.

SYMPTOMS

Insulin shock, which can come on suddenly, can cause any or all of the following symptoms:

- Hunger
- Pale and sweaty skin
- Excited and/or sometimes belligerent behavior
- Shallow breathing

WHAT TO DO

If the victim is conscious:
1. Give the victim food containing sugar, such as fruit juice, sweetened drinks, honey, or just sugar in water.
2. Seek medical attention immediately.

If the victim is unconscious:
Seek medical attention promptly, preferably at the nearest hospital emergency department.

SEPTIC SHOCK

Septic shock is a life-threatening condition in which the body's tissues and vital organs are unable to use nutrients from the blood. This form of shock is brought on by an infection in the bloodstream, usually caused by bacteria.

SYMPTOMS

Septic shock can cause any or all of the following symptoms:

- Sudden fever
- Vomiting

- Light-headedness or dizziness
- Fainting
- Weakness

WHAT TO DO

1. Call 911 (or your local emergency number) or take the person immediately to the nearest hospital emergency department.
2. Maintain an open airway. Restore breathing and circulation if necessary. (See pp. 31–50.)
3. Keep the victim lying down.
4. Cover the victim only enough to prevent loss of body heat. Keep the victim comfortable.

STREPTOCOCCAL TOXIC SHOCK–LIKE SYNDROME

Streptococcal toxic shock–like syndrome is a severe infection that is fatal in about a third of the people who develop it. The infection is caused by a virulent form of streptococcal bacteria sometimes referred to as "flesh-eating bacteria." The infection usually occurs in otherwise healthy people between ages 20 and 50 and, for unknown reasons, may result from a sore throat or a minor injury to the skin.

SYMPTOMS

Streptococcal toxic shock–like syndrome can cause any or all of the following symptoms:

- Sudden fever
- Shaking chills
- Muscle pain
- Confusion
- Fast heart rate
- Pain in the arms or legs
- Vomiting
- Headache
- Mild redness of the skin or a localized rash that may progress into blisters or develop a bluish color

WHAT TO DO

1. Call 911 (or your local emergency number) or take the person immediately to the nearest hospital emergency department.
2. Maintain an open airway. Restore breathing and circulation if necessary. (See pp. 31–50.)
3. Keep the victim lying down.
4. Cover the victim only enough to prevent loss of body heat. Keep the victim comfortable.

TOXIC SHOCK SYNDROME

Toxic shock is a serious, rare infection caused by staphylococcal bacteria. Toxins produced by the bacteria enter the bloodstream and are spread throughout the body. As in other forms of shock, toxic shock restricts the supply of oxygenated blood from reaching body tissues, which can be fatal.

The infection was previously associated primarily with the use of high-absorbency tampons (which have now been taken off the market). Most cases now result from packing around wounds (such as nosebleeds) that become infected for unknown reasons.

SYMPTOMS

Toxic shock syndrome can cause any or all of the following symptoms:

- Sudden fever
- Vomiting and/or diarrhea
- Light-headedness or dizziness
- Aching muscles and joints
- Headache
- Weak pulse
- Fainting
- Weakness
- Rash, similar to a sunburn, that may spread to the palms of the hands and soles of the feet in about a week (skin looks like it is peeling)

WHAT TO DO

1. Call 911 (or your local emergency number) or take the person immediately to the nearest hospital emergency department.

INJURIES AND ILLNESSES

Maintain an open airway. Restore breathing and circulation if necessary. (See pp. 31–50.)

2. Keep the victim lying down.
3. Cover the victim only enough to prevent loss of body heat. Keep the victim comfortable.

See Also: Bites and Stings (Insect Stings), p. 73; Bleeding, p. 96; Drug Abuse, p. 156; Electrical Burns, p. 168; Heart Attack, p. 204; Seizures, p. 237; Unconsciousness, p. 259; Wounds, p. 264.

SPLINTERS

A splinter, or sliver, is a small piece of wood, glass, or other material that becomes lodged under the surface of the skin.

WHAT TO DO

1. Wash your hands and the victim's skin around the splinter with soap and water.
2. Place a sewing needle and tweezers in boiling water for about 5 minutes or hold over an open flame to sterilize.
3. If the splinter is sticking out of the skin, gently pull the splinter out with the tweezers at the same angle at which it entered.
4. If the splinter is not deeply lodged beneath the skin and is clearly visible, gently loosen the skin around the splinter with the needle and carefully remove the splinter with the tweezers at the same angle at which it entered. Make sure you remove the entire splinter.
5. Squeeze the wound gently to allow slight bleeding to wash out any germs. Or rinse out the wound under running water for at least 5 minutes.
6. If the splinter breaks off in the skin, is easily broken, or is deeply lodged, seek medical attention for removal and a possible tetanus shot. You should also seek medical attention for any damage to a nail.
7. After the splinter is removed, wash the area with soap and water and apply a bandage.
8. Watch for any signs of infection such as redness, pus, or red streaks leading up the body from the wound; see a doctor immediately if you notice any of these symptoms.

See Also: Bleeding, p. 96.

SPRAINS

A sprain is an injury to the ligaments—strong, flexible bands of fibrous tissue that bind bones together and support the joints. A ligament may be stretched or completely torn. A sprain usually results from overextending or twisting a limb beyond its normal range of movement.

SYMPTOMS

A sprain can cause any or all of the following symptoms:

- A popping sound or tearing sensation at the time of the injury
- Pain on moving the injured part and/or pain in the joint
- Swelling of the joint
- Tenderness on touching the affected area
- Black and blue discoloration of skin around the area of the injury

WHAT TO DO

If you are uncertain about whether an injury is a sprain or a broken bone, treat it as a broken bone. (See Broken Bones, p. 107.)

If the ankle or knee is sprained:
1. Place cold packs or a small ice bag wrapped in a cloth over the affected area intermittently (30 minutes on, 30 minutes off) for the first 12 to 24 hours to decrease swelling. *Do not* use heat or hot water soaks during the first 24 hours following the injury.
2. Apply a supporting bandage, pillow, or blanket splint to the injury. (See Splinting and Other Procedures, p. 109.) Loosen the support if the swelling increases.
3. Keep the injured part elevated above the level of the heart and keep the victim from walking if possible.
4. After the first 24 hours, apply heat to the area or soak it in warm water periodically for several minutes at a time.

5. Seek medical attention for an evaluation of the injury and to rule out a broken bone.

If the wrist, elbow, or shoulder is sprained:
1. Place the injured arm in a sling. For a wrist injury, apply a supporting bandage. Loosen the bandage if swelling increases. (See Bandages, p. 23.)
2. Place cold packs or a small ice bag wrapped in a cloth over the affected area. *Do not* use heat or hot water soaks during the first 24 hours following the injury.
3. Seek medical attention for an evaluation of the injury and to rule out a broken bone.

See Also: Broken Bones, p. 107; Dislocations, p. 151; Muscle Aches and Pains, p. 220; Sports First Aid, pp. 271–336.

INJURIES AND ILLNESSES

A stroke results from an interruption in blood flow to part or all of the brain. This interruption in circulation may be caused by the formation of a clot inside an artery supplying blood to the brain, by a clot elsewhere in the body that blocks the blood supply to the brain, by narrowing of a blood vessel, or by bursting of an artery within the brain. The brain must receive adequate amounts of blood to function properly. The sooner the victim of a stroke receives treatment, the more successful treatment is likely to be in preventing or reversing any brain damage.

MAJOR STROKE

SYMPTOMS

A major stroke can cause any or all of the following symptoms:

- Sudden headache
- Sudden paralysis, weakness, or numbness on one side of the body; the corner of the mouth may droop
- Loss or slurring of speech
- Possible unconsciousness or mental confusion
- Sudden fall
- Impaired vision or double vision
- Pupils of different size
- Incoordination
- Difficulty breathing, chewing, talking, and/or swallowing
- Loss of bladder and/or bowel control
- Strong, slow pulse

WHAT TO DO

1. Call 911 (or your local emergency number) or take the person to the nearest emergency department immediately. The sooner treatment is begun, the more successful it is likely to be.

2. Maintain an open airway. Restore breathing and circulation if necessary. (See pp. 31–50.)
3. Place the victim on his or her weak side so that secretions can drain from the mouth. *Do not* give fluids or food to the victim. He or she may vomit or choke on them.
4. Keep the victim comfortably warm and quiet. Reassure and calm the victim.
5. Apply cold cloths to the victim's head.

TRANSIENT ISCHEMIC ATTACK

A transient ischemic attack (TIA) is a spasm of a blood vessel in the brain. Symptoms usually occur in people between the ages of 50 and 70 and usually clear up within 24 hours.

SYMPTOMS

A TIA can cause any or all of the following symptoms:

• Slight mental confusion
• Slight dizziness
• Minor speech difficulties
• Muscle weakness

WHAT TO DO

1. Call 911 (or your local emergency number) or take the person to the nearest emergency department immediately. The sooner treatment is begun, the more successful it is likely to be.
2. Maintain an open airway. Restore breathing and circulation if necessary. (See pp. 31–50.)
3. Place the victim on his or her weak side so that secretions can drain from the mouth. *Do not* give fluids or food to the victim. He or she may vomit or choke on them.
4. Keep the victim comfortably warm and quiet. Reassure and calm the victim.
5. Apply cold cloths to the victim's head.

INJURIES AND ILLNESSES

SUICIDE, THREATENED

Take all threats of suicide seriously—even though you cannot imagine that a person could be feeling so unhappy that he or she would want to die. A person who threatens to take his or her life sees the situation as hopeless and death as the only answer. Your response could make the difference between life and death—a person who is contemplating suicide very often changes his or her mind when given the chance. You can provide that chance by diverting the person's attention from immediate thoughts of self-destruction.

If the threat of suicide is unmistakable and immediate:
1. Immediately phone for help; call 911 (or your local emergency number), a suicide hotline, the police, or other trained professionals.
2. De-escalate the situation. Even though you may feel very nervous, speak calmly and move slowly. Sometimes a suicidal person is feeling very angry and may lash out at those who are closest. Do not argue with the person or show anger; these actions could intensify the situation.
3. Give the person your full attention. Try to get him or her to talk to you, but don't insist. Simply being there and showing a willingness to respond when the person is ready to talk can be very reassuring. You may find it difficult to sit without talking, but even your silent presence can be very soothing to a person who is suicidal. When he or she chooses to open up and talk to you, listen attentively. It is OK to sympathize with the person's feelings; showing that you understand can make him or her feel less alone.
4. Once the immediate, critical situation is under control, seek professional help for the person. If possible, you or someone else the person trusts should go along to the therapy sessions.

If the person is talking about suicide but does not have the means at hand:

1. Remain calm, listen attentively, or simply sit silently with the person. Although the immediate situation is not critical, it is still extremely serious.
2. Get the person to agree to get help from a medical professional as soon as possible; call your doctor and ask him or her to recommend a qualified professional. If you would feel better getting immediate help, take the person to an emergency department or counseling center right away.
3. Remove or lock away any firearms or medications (including over-the-counter drugs).
4. If possible, prevent the person from driving.
5. If the person refuses to seek help, call 911 (or your local emergency number) or a suicide hotline immediately for help. Don't be concerned about overreacting—you will feel better than if you find out later that you could have helped and didn't.

SIGNS TO WATCH FOR IN AN ADULT

There are no clear-cut ways to tell in advance who will succeed at suicide and who won't. Always err on the side of safety and seek professional help if you suspect a person may be suicidal. The following signs may indicate that an adult is at risk of committing suicide:

- Severe depression that lasts longer than a few weeks and is characterized by symptoms that can include loss of appetite, a change in sleep patterns (sleeping less than usual or more than usual), and lack of interest in formerly enjoyable activities
- Excessive drinking or abuse of other drugs
- A previous suicide attempt
- A history of suicide in the family
- Giving away or selling valuable possessions
- Recent filing of a will
- Failure to renew a rental lease or other indications that the person is not thinking about the future

SIGNS TO WATCH FOR IN A CHILD

The signs of depression and suicide risk are different in children than in adults. A suicide threat by a child is extremely serious be-

INJURIES AND ILLNESSES

cause children do not have the same judgment as adults and don't always understand the consequences of their actions. A child who talks about suicide should not be left alone until he or she has had a thorough evaluation by a mental health professional, preferably a child psychiatrist. Call your doctor or a suicide hotline immediately if you notice any of the following signs in a child. Even if the child is not suicidal, these are indications that he or she has a physical or emotional problem that requires the attention of a physician:

- An obvious change in behavior such as worsening performance in school, withdrawal from friends and family, change in sleep patterns or appetite, or lack of interest in formerly enjoyable activities
- Anger that may be displayed in disruptive, unmanageable behavior or physical violence against other children or adults
- Irritability
- Moodiness
- Use of alcohol or other drugs

Sunburn is usually a first-degree burn of the skin resulting from overexposure to the sun. Prolonged exposure can lead to a second-degree burn. The peak hours for sunburn, when the ultraviolet rays from the sun are most harmful, are between 10 AM and 3 PM.

SYMPTOMS

Sunburn can cause any or all of the following symptoms, which usually subside in 2 or 3 days:

- Redness
- Pain
- Mild swelling
- Blisters and swelling in severe cases
- Itching

WHAT TO DO

1. Put cold water on the sunburned area.
2. If sunburn is severe, submerge the sunburned area under cold water until pain is relieved. It is also helpful to place cold, wet cloths on the burned area. Do not rub the skin. Taking ibuprofen may help reduce pain and redness.
3. Elevate severely sunburned arms or legs.
4. If possible, put a dry, sterile bandage on a severely sunburned area.
5. Seek medical attention for severe sunburn. *Do not* break blisters or put ointments, sprays, antiseptic medications, or home remedies on severe sunburns.

INJURIES AND ILLNESSES

255

Preventing Sunburn

Here are some steps you can take to avoid sunburn:

- Wear protective clothing such as long sleeves and a wide-brim hat.
- If you have light skin, wear a sunscreen with a sun protection factor (SPF) of at least 15 for routine activities and 25 to 30 for prolonged outdoor activity. If your skin is darker, wear a sunscreen with an SPF of 6 or 8 for routine activities and at least 15 for prolonged outdoor activity. Blocking agents such as zinc and iron oxide are also effective at blocking radiation.

See Also: Burns, p. 121; Dehydration, p. 145; Fever, p. 180; Seizures, p. 237.

TOOTH PROBLEMS

TOOTHACHE

Cavities and infections often cause toothaches. Home treatment offers only temporary relief from pain but is often helpful if a toothache occurs in the middle of the night or before you can seek professional attention. A trip to the dentist is necessary to find the exact cause of a toothache and to treat it effectively.

WHAT TO DO

1. Give the victim aspirin, acetaminophen, naproxen, or ibuprofen. Aspirin should be swallowed and not applied directly to the affected area. Do not give aspirin to a child under 16 years because of the risk of Reye's syndrome, a life-threatening condition that has been linked to aspirin.
2. Place cold compresses or ice packs on the face over the affected area. For some people, warm compresses may be more comforting. This varies with each individual.
3. Seek dental attention.

KNOCKED-OUT TOOTH

A tooth that has been knocked out can be successfully reimplanted in the gum within 30 minutes of the injury. You can purchase a tooth-preservation kit at most drugstores to keep on hand; bring it along whenever you or your children are participating in sports activities.

WHAT TO DO

1. Rinse the tooth gently in cool water (don't use soap), and hold it in place in the socket with a clean washcloth or piece of gauze, or put it in a clean container with some milk or saliva,

which will keep the tooth alive until the dentist reimplants it. *Do not* put the tooth in tap water. The minerals in water may cause further harm. Saline (salt) water may be used, however.

2. If bleeding is present, fold a clean piece of gauze, handkerchief, or tissue into a pad and place it over the wound. Close teeth tightly to apply firm pressure to the bleeding area. Maintain pressure for 20 to 30 minutes. Repeat the procedure if necessary.

3. Take the victim and the tooth to the dentist or hospital emergency department immediately.

TOOTH EXTRACTION

Pain, slight swelling, and bleeding often occur after a tooth has been pulled. If these problems become severe or persistent, consult your dentist.

WHAT TO DO

1. As soon as possible after the tooth has been pulled, place a cold compress or ice bag on the face on the affected area to relieve swelling. The compress should remain in place for 15 minutes out of each hour. Repeat the procedure for several hours.

2. If bleeding is present, fold a clean piece of gauze, handkerchief, or tissue into a pad and place it over the wound. Close teeth tightly to apply firm pressure to the bleeding area. Maintain pressure for 20 to 30 minutes. Repeat the procedure if necessary.

3. If the dentist did not prescribe medication for pain, acetaminophen, naproxen, or ibuprofen may be taken. Aspirin should not be taken because it can increase bleeding.

See Also: Head, Neck, and Back Injuries, p. 194.

UNCONSCIOUSNESS

There are many causes of unconsciousness including heart attack, stroke, head injury, bleeding, diabetic coma, or insulin shock. Poisoning, heatstroke, choking, gas inhalation, severe allergic reaction to insect stings, and electrical burns can also cause unconsciousness. You should always seek medical attention for anyone who is unconscious, regardless of the cause.

SYMPTOMS

A person who is unconscious is:

• Unresponsive
• Unaware of his or her surroundings

WHAT TO DO

1. Call 911 (or your local emergency number).
2. Restore breathing and circulation if necessary. (See pp. 31–50.)

If the unconscious victim is breathing:
1. Call 911 (or your local emergency number) or take the person to the nearest emergency department.
2. Maintain an open airway.
3. Loosen tight clothing, particularly around the victim's neck. Keep the victim comfortably warm but not hot. *Do not* give an unconscious victim anything to eat or drink and *do not* leave him or her alone.
4. Keep the victim lying down. If the cause of unconsciousness is unknown, always suspect a head, neck, or back injury and do not move the victim except to maintain an open airway. If the cause of unconsciousness is known and it is not a head, neck, or back injury, place the victim on his or her side to allow se-

cretions to drain and to prevent choking on fluids and vomit. When placed on his or her side, the victim should have the head slightly lower than the rest of the body.

5. Check for bleeding (p. 96), broken bones (p. 107), or a head injury (p. 194), and give first aid.

VERTIGO

Vertigo is a disturbance in the balance mechanism of the inner ear. This disturbance may be caused by an ear infection, an allergy, injury to the inner ear, or decreased blood flow to the head.

SYMPTOMS

Vertigo can cause any or all of the following symptoms:

- Loss of balance
- Dizziness (feeling that everything is spinning around or that the person is spinning around)
- Nausea with or without vomiting

WHAT TO DO

1. Reassure the person that he or she is not turning or spinning around.
2. Assist the person so that he or she does not fall.
3. Seek medical attention.

INJURIES AND ILLNESSES

VOMITING

Vomiting may occur with many conditions. It is particularly common with viral infections of the intestines, excessive eating, excessive drinking, and emotional upsets. Vomiting may also be present with more serious conditions such as asthma, animal bites, allergic reactions to insect stings or bites, heart attack, heat exhaustion, shock due to injuries, food poisoning, and head injuries.

Vomiting associated with intestinal viruses, excessive eating or drinking, and emotional stress usually does not last long. Any vomiting, however, that is severe or lasts longer than a day or two needs medical attention because dehydration (loss of body fluids) or a chemical imbalance (loss of body chemicals) can occur—especially in infants, the elderly, or people who have a chronic illness.

Vomiting can indicate a serious problem. Always seek medical attention promptly if vomiting occurs with severe stomach pain or after a recent head injury, or if the vomit contains blood that looks like coffee grounds.

WHAT TO DO

To treat simple vomiting associated with intestinal upsets, replace lost fluids by frequently sipping liquids such as carbonated beverages (shaken up to eliminate the fizz), juice, or bouillon. After vomiting has stopped, avoid solid food. Work slowly back to a regular diet.

If a person is unconscious and vomiting, he or she should be placed on his or her side with the head extended to prevent choking on vomit. Do this only if there is no head, neck, or back injury. A person with a head injury should have his or her head turned to the side to prevent choking. Do this very carefully by rolling the person over as a unit, keeping his or her head in the same line with the rest of the body as you found it (see p. 194).

VOMITING IN INFANTS AND YOUNG CHILDREN

Vomiting in infants and children is common. Some of the most frequent causes include allergy, viral infections (flu), poisoning, car sickness, intestinal obstructions, pneumonia, colic, or head injuries.

In newborns and infants, spitting up food after eating is common and is *not* the same as vomiting. It is usually not serious as long as the infant is not choking.

You should always talk to the doctor any time a child under 2 years is vomiting. Vomiting in infants can be quite serious, particularly if vomited material is expelled with such force that it shoots out of the infant's mouth 1 or 2 feet across the room (projectile vomiting). This type of vomiting always needs prompt medical attention. It could represent a partially or completely obstructed intestine.

Prolonged vomiting or vomiting with diarrhea can lead to dehydration (loss of body fluids) and also needs prompt medical attention. Other possibly serious symptoms to watch for in infants and small children include vomit that contains blood, and vomiting with fever, headache, or stomachache.

WHAT TO DO

To treat simple vomiting that accompanies intestinal upsets, give the child fluids and avoid solid foods. Give small sips (approximately 1 teaspoon) of a pediatric rehydrating solution or water every 10 to 20 minutes. Gradually increase the amount if the child is keeping the fluids down. Slowly work back to a regular diet once the child's stomach is settled.

See Also: Abdominal Pain, p. 59; Bites and Stings, p. 72; Cold-Related Problems, p. 139; Diarrhea, p. 148; Drug Abuse, p. 156; Food Poisoning, p. 185; Heat-Related Problems, p. 206.

OPEN WOUNDS

An open wound is an injury in which the skin is broken. The objectives in treating an open wound consist of:

- Stopping the bleeding.
- Preventing contamination and infection.
- Preventing shock.
- Seeking medical attention if the wound is severe or if the victim has not had a tetanus shot within 5 years.

Abdominal Wounds

Deep abdominal wounds are a medical emergency. Surgery is usually necessary to repair the wound.

WHAT TO DO

1. Call 911 (or your local emergency number) or take the person to the nearest emergency department.
2. Maintain an open airway. Restore breathing and circulation if necessary. (See pp. 31–50.)
3. Keep the victim lying down on his or her back.
4. Bend the victim's legs at the knees and place a pillow, rolled towel, blanket, or clothing under his or her knees to relax the abdominal muscles.
5. Apply direct pressure to the abdomen if necessary to control bleeding. (See Internal Bleeding, p. 100.) The abdomen is soft and applying pressure can decrease or stop internal bleeding.
6. *Do not* try to push the intestines back in place if they are sticking out of the wound. If medical assistance is not readily available and the intestine is sticking out of the wound, dampen a pad with sterile or boiled water that has cooled to body tem-

perature (drinking water or clean seawater may be used in an emergency) and place the pad over the intestine.

7. Cover the *entire* wound with a sterile pad such as gauze (preferably) or a clean cloth, clothing, towel, plastic wrap, aluminum foil, or other suitable material.

8. Apply an adhesive bandage to hold the pad in place. Do not bandage too tightly.

9. Keep the victim comfortably warm. *Do not* give the victim anything to eat or drink, including water, as surgery will probably be necessary and the stomach should be empty.

Chest Wounds

A deep, open chest wound is a serious emergency. Damage to the lungs may occur, resulting in air flowing in and out of the wound with breathing and not in and out of the lungs where it is needed.

WHAT TO DO

1. Call 911 (or your local emergency number).

2. *Do not* remove any object remaining in the wound, as *very* serious bleeding or other internal life-threatening problems may result.

3. Immediately cover the *entire* wound and about 2 inches all around it with a pad, such as dry sterile gauze (preferably), a clean cloth, clothing, plastic wrap, aluminum foil, or other suitable material. The pad *must* be at least 2 inches larger all around the wound and must be airtight.

4. If no pad is available, place a hand on each side of the wound and firmly push the skin together to close the wound. Apply an airtight bandage with tape or other suitable material if available.

5. Maintain an open airway. Restore breathing and circulation if necessary. (See pp. 31–50.) It may be necessary to slightly raise the victim's shoulders to aid breathing.

6. *Do not* give the victim anything to eat or drink, as this may cause choking. Also, the stomach should be empty in case surgery is necessary.

7. Reassure the victim. Gentleness, kindness, and understanding play an important role in treating a victim who may be in shock.

INJURIES AND ILLNESSES

Cuts

WHAT TO DO

If bleeding is severe:
Use direct pressure to control bleeding. (See External Bleeding, p. 96.)

If bleeding is not severe:
1. Wash your hands thoroughly with soap and water before handling the wound to prevent further contamination of the injury.
2. If the cut is still bleeding, apply direct pressure over the wound with a sterile or clean cloth.
3. When the bleeding has stopped, wash the wound thoroughly with soap and water to remove any dirt or other foreign material near the skin's surface. Gentle scrubbing may be necessary. It is very important to remove all dirt to prevent infection. Foreign particles close to the skin's surface may be carefully removed with tweezers that have been sterilized over an open flame or boiled in water. *Do not* attempt to remove any foreign material that is deeply embedded in a muscle or other tissue, as serious bleeding may result.
4. Rinse the wound thoroughly under running water for 5 to 10 minutes.
5. Pat the wound dry with a sterile or clean cloth. *Do not* apply ointments, medication, antiseptic spray, or home remedies unless told to do so by a doctor.
6. Cover the wound with a sterile dressing and tape it in place. If the cut is slightly gaping, apply a butterfly bandage (see p. 24) or tape the edges of the wound together as close as possible.
7. Always seek medical attention if:
   • The wound is severe.
   • Bleeding does not stop.
   • The injury was caused by an obviously dirty object.
   • The wound was caused by an animal or human bite.
   • A foreign material or object is embedded in the wound.
   • You notice signs of infection such as fever, redness, swelling, increased tenderness at the site of the wound, pus, or red streaks leading from the wound toward the body.
   • There is any doubt about the victim having had a tetanus immunization within 5 years.

8. If medical assistance is not readily available and the wound shows signs of infection, keep the victim lying down with the injured area immobilized and elevated. Apply warm wet cloths over the wound until medical assistance can be obtained.

Cuts in the Scalp

Cuts in the scalp may bleed heavily even if the wound is minor. *With any cut or puncture, you should consult a physician about the necessity for a tetanus shot.*

WHAT TO DO

If the cut is severe or there is the possibility of a skull fracture:
1. *Do not* clean the wound or remove any foreign bodies from the scalp.
2. Gently apply a sterile compress and bandage it in place. If bleeding persists, apply pressure firmly to the wound until the bleeding stops.
3. Seek medical attention promptly.

If the cut is minor:
1. Control the bleeding by applying a sterile compress to the wound and pressing firmly.
2. When bleeding stops, clean the wound with soap and water or hydrogen peroxide.
3. Apply a bandage.

Puncture Wounds

A puncture wound results when a sharp object—such as a nail, a large splinter, a knife, a needle, a bullet, a firecracker, or an ice pick—pierces the skin and underlying tissue. The wound is usually deep and narrow, with little bleeding, which increases the chance for infection because the germs are not washed out by the flow of blood.

Tetanus is a danger with any wound, but is greater with puncture wounds since the tetanus bacteria grow well in a deep wound where there is little oxygen. *All* puncture injuries should be seen by a doctor.

INJURIES AND ILLNESSES

1. Wash your hands with soap and water before examining the wound.
2. *Do not* poke or put medication into the wound. Look to see if any part of the object that caused the injury has broken off and become lodged in the wound. *Do not* attempt to remove any foreign object that is deeply embedded in the wound, as the foreign object may break off in the wound and serious bleeding may result.
3. In obviously minor puncture wounds, objects sticking in no deeper than the skin's surface may be carefully removed with tweezers that have been sterilized over an open flame or boiled in water.
4. Encourage bleeding to wash out germs from inside the wound by gently pressing on the edge of the wound. *Do not* press so hard that you cause additional injury to the wound.
5. If the puncture wound is obviously minor, wash the wound with soap and water and rinse it under running water.
6. Cover the wound with a sterile or clean dressing and bandage it in place.
7. Seek medical attention promptly.
8. If medical attention is not readily available and the wound shows signs of infection—such as fever, redness, swelling, increased tenderness at the site of the wound, pus, or red streaks leading from the wound toward the body—keep the victim lying down with the injured area immobilized and elevated. Apply warm wet cloths to the wound until medical assistance can be obtained.

Scrapes and Scratches

Scrapes can easily become infected since the outer, protective skin layer is destroyed.

1. Wash your hands with soap and water before treating the wound.
2. Wash the injured area well with soap and water to remove any dirt. Gentle scrubbing may be necessary. It is important to remove all dirt to prevent infection. Bits of dirt left in the wound

may also cause permanent discoloration of the skin. Rinse the wound under running water. *Do not* put medication on the wound unless a doctor recommends it.

3. Leave minor scrapes and scratches exposed to the air. Cover larger wounds, or those likely to be reinjured, with a sterile pad or clean cloth and tape it in place.

4. If you notice any signs of infection—such as redness, swelling, increased tenderness at the site of the wound, pus, or red streaks leading from the wound toward the body—keep the victim lying down with the injured area immobilized and elevated. Apply warm wet cloths to the wound and seek medical assistance immediately.

5. You should also seek medical attention if the wound is large or deep or there is a question about the victim having had a tetanus immunization within 5 years.

INJURIES AND ILLNESSES

PART III

SPORTS

FIRST

AID

The ankle consists of the bones of the lower leg (the fibula and tibia) and the top of the foot (the talus). These bones form the ankle joint and are connected by a group of ligaments. Two important ligaments that help add stability to the joint are the anterior talofibular ligament, which runs from the outer ankle "knob" to the top of the foot, and the calcaneofibular ligament, which connects the outer ankle knob to the heel bone. The ankle is a hinge joint that allows up-and-down bending and limited side-to-side movement of the foot.

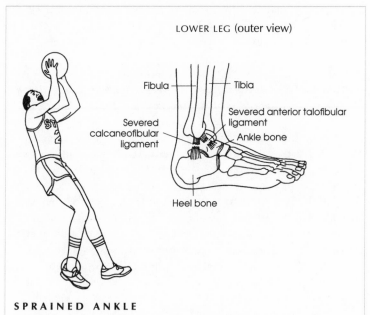

LOWER LEG (outer view)

Fibula — | — Tibia

Severed anterior talofibular ligament

Severed calcaneofibular ligament

Ankle bone

Heel bone

SPRAINED ANKLE

A sprained ankle is an injury to one or both ligaments on the outside of the ankle. The injury results from stepping down on the outside of the foot (see following pages).

SPORTS FIRST AID

273

SPRAINED ANKLE

A sprained ankle occurs when a person steps down on the outside of the foot, causing the ligaments on the outside of the ankle to stretch or tear. The injury, which may involve one or both ligaments, can range from a tiny tear to complete severing of the ligaments. A sprained ankle can be more painful than a break in a bone and may take as long to heal. Sprained ankles are the most common injuries in all sports, including baseball, basketball, football, soccer, rugby, jogging, track and field, and tennis, and can also occur during everyday activities, including walking.

SYMPTOMS

At the time of the injury, you may feel a flash of heat or a tearing sensation on the outside of the ankle or hear a popping sound. Pain, swelling, and bruising may develop on the outside of the ankle or the top of the foot and you will not be able to walk on it. Your ankle may feel warm for several hours. Depending on the severity of the sprain, symptoms may appear immediately or 6 to 12 hours after the injury.

Immediate Treatment *If the pain is severe or persistent or if your ankle is swollen, see your physician to determine proper treatment. He or she can rule out a broken bone in the foot, ankle, or lower leg.*

Stop the activity that caused the sprain. As soon as possible, place an ice pack on the ankle intermittently (20 minutes every hour while you're awake) for the first 24 to 48 hours after the injury. Cold treatments help stop internal bleeding and the accumulation of fluids in and around the injured area, thereby decreasing swelling. Elevate your ankle above the level of your heart.

Unless your doctor has prescribed another medication, take aspirin, ibuprofen, naproxen, or ketoprofen as directed to relieve pain and inflammation. (Acetaminophen relieves pain but has no effect against inflammation; ask your doctor or pharmacist for guidance.)

> **WARNING**
>
> MEDICATIONS
>
> Take the following precautions with medications:
>
> • If you are allergic to aspirin or if you have a history of peptic ulcers, you should not take ibuprofen, naproxen, or ketoprofen; ask your doctor about this.
> • Do not drink alcohol if you are taking aspirin, acetaminophen, ibuprofen, naproxen, or ketoprofen; combining these painkillers with alcohol increases the risk of liver damage or stomach bleeding.
> • If you are pregnant or nursing, talk to your doctor before taking any medication, even one sold over the counter.
> • Never give aspirin to a child under 18 years because the drug is linked to a life-threatening condition called Reye's syndrome in children.

Continued Care Do not engage in the activity that caused the injury until the pain has subsided. Your physician may put a brace on the ankle to immobilize or restrict movement. Occasional use of an elastic bandage on the ankle may aid stability. (If you have peripheral vascular disease or diabetes, consult your physician first before using an elastic bandage.) Take aspirin, ibuprofen, naproxen, or ketoprofen as directed to relieve pain and inflammation. See your physician if the pain and swelling continue.

Once an ankle has been sprained, it may be susceptible to recurring sprains because of instability in the joint. Swelling and the development of bone spurs (small, spokelike calcium growths) can make the ankle susceptible to arthritis.

How to Prevent Recurring Injury Wear properly fitting shoes that are appropriate for the activity and replace them when they wear out. You may have to tape your ankle to make it more stable. With your physician's okay, work with a trainer or physical therapist to strengthen the muscles around the ankle and lower calf.

SPORTS FIRST AID

The lower back consists of the vertebrae and discs of the lower spine, the sacrum and coccyx (tailbone), and many muscles and ligaments that connect the chest wall to the pelvis. The spine and muscles provide support for the trunk and protect the spinal cord.

LOWER BACK PAIN

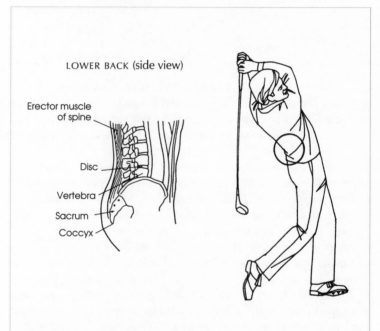

LOWER BACK (side view)

Erector muscle of spine

Disc

Vertebra

Sacrum

Coccyx

LOWER BACK PAIN

Lower back pain can occur for a variety of reasons including a strain or tear in a muscle or ligament, injury to a disc or vertebra, pressure on a nerve, or fatigue. Over time, a repetitive motion such as a golf swing can also bring on lower back pain.

Lower back pain can occur for a variety of reasons: a strain or tear in a muscle or ligament, injury to a disc or vertebra, pressure on a nerve, or fatigue. Lower back pain can be caused by a repetitive motion, such as a golf swing over time, or by a sudden force exerted on the back, such as from a football block. It can also result from an insufficient warm-up period before athletic activity.

SYMPTOMS

Symptoms can range from a dull ache to a sharp pain in the lower back. If a muscle tears, you may feel a slight pull when the injury occurs, with pain intensifying several hours after the injury. A herniated disc may produce sharp pains that make movement difficult. Sciatic nerve damage may produce sharp pains that radiate down the back of one or both legs. A back that is fatigued, such as from a long-distance athletic activity, may be stiff and ache all over.

Immediate Treatment *See your physician if your back pain is caused by a blow to the back, if the pain is severe or radiates down the back of both legs, if you have numbness or tingling in your lower back or legs, or if the pain gets worse when you cough or sneeze. Go to the nearest hospital emergency department if you suddenly have problems holding urine or controlling bowel movements or if you have sudden and noticeable weakness in your legs.*

For muscle pulls or tears, place an ice pack on the area intermittently (20 minutes every hour while you're awake) for the first 24 to 48 hours after the injury. Cold treatments help stop internal bleeding and the accumulation of fluids in and around the injured area, thereby decreasing swelling.

For stiffness or fatigue, place a heating pad on the back to help relax the muscles. Soreness in the lower back can also be relieved by lying down, which takes pressure off the back; by placing one foot on a foot rest when you're standing, which shifts the angle of the sacrum, lessening the arch of the back; or by getting a good night's rest.

Unless your doctor has prescribed another medication, take aspirin, ibuprofen, naproxen, or ketoprofen as directed. (Acetaminophen may not contain as much of the anti-inflammatory agents as aspirin, ibuprofen, naproxen, or ketoprofen; ask your doctor or pharmacist for guidance.)

SPORTS FIRST AID

277

>
> ## WARNING
>
> MEDICATIONS
>
> Here are some precautions to take with medications:
>
> - If you are allergic to aspirin, you may also be allergic to ibuprofen, naproxen, or ketoprofen; ask your doctor about this.
> - Do not drink alcohol if you are taking aspirin, acetaminophen, ibuprofen, naproxen, or ketoprofen; combining these painkillers with alcohol increases the risk of liver damage or stomach bleeding.
> - If you are pregnant or nursing, talk to your doctor before taking any medication, even one sold over the counter.
> - Never give aspirin to a child under 18 years because the drug is linked to a life-threatening condition called Reye's syndrome in children.

Continued Care For a muscle pull or tear, place an ice pack on the injury at least once a day for 2 to 4 days. Thereafter, use a heating pad on your back at least once a day until the injury heals. Use a heating pad thereafter. Heat increases blood circulation in the area, providing vital nutrients to the injury and helping speed recovery. *Do not* apply heat before the swelling has subsided, or swelling in the injured area may increase. Take aspirin, ibuprofen, naproxen, or ketoprofen as directed to reduce pain and inflammation.

Avoid athletic activity until the injury has had time to heal or until the pain is gone. The length of time that it takes the injury to heal depends on the type and severity of the injury, and can range from 3 to 6 weeks or longer. Once the injury has healed, gradually and carefully do exercises that stretch the muscles in your back. Use an ice pack to reduce any swelling that may occur, and, after the swelling has subsided, apply heat to help relax the injured muscle. See your physician if the pain continues or recurs. With proper rest, lower back pain usually has no long-term effects.

For stiffness or fatigue, apply heat as directed under Immediate Treatment (p. 277).

How to Prevent Recurring Injury Work with a trainer or physical therapist on exercises that strengthen the muscles in your back and abdomen. Stretch the muscles in your back before engaging in sports. Avoid sudden movements that could reinjure your back.

The elbow is a hinge joint that allows the wrist and hand to rotate and the forearm to extend and flex. The elbow consists of three main bones—the humerus of the upper arm and the ulna and radius of the forearm—that converge to form the elbow joint. The bony protrusions on the inside and outside of the elbow are called epicondyles. Ligaments connect and support the three bones in the elbow. Tendons are strong, flexible cords that connect the surrounding muscles to the bones. Bursas—fluid-filled sacs or saclike cavities—surround and cushion the bones at the joint.

ELBOW BURSITIS

Elbow bursitis (sometimes referred to as student's elbow or miner's elbow) is inflammation and swelling of the olecranon bursa, a fluid-filled sac at the base of the elbow, beneath the ulna bone in the forearm. The bursa (which lies just under the skin) cushions the bones at the joint and allows the skin to glide smoothly over the muscles and tendons of the outer elbow. The condition results from repetitive stress (such as from leaning on the point of the elbow for long, frequent intervals) or from a direct blow (such as from a fall).

SYMPTOMS

Elbow bursitis usually causes a painless swelling about the size of a golf ball on the outer elbow. Unless the swelling is severe, the condition usually does not affect the elbow's range of motion.

Immediate Treatment *If the swelling is painful, if your skin at the site of the swelling is warm or red, or if you have a fever, see your physician to determine proper treatment.*

Rest the elbow in a splint or an elastic wrap bandage until the swelling subsides. Unless your doctor has prescribed another

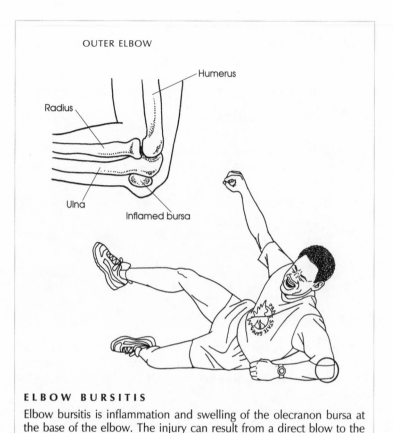

OUTER ELBOW

Radius

Humerus

Ulna

Inflamed bursa

ELBOW BURSITIS

Elbow bursitis is inflammation and swelling of the olecranon bursa at the base of the elbow. The injury can result from a direct blow to the elbow, such as from a fall.

medication, take aspirin, ibuprofen, naproxen, or ketoprofen as directed to relieve pain and inflammation. (Acetaminophen relieves pain but has no effect against inflammation; ask your doctor or pharmacist for guidance.) For a recurring case, your doctor may recommend an injection of a corticosteroid drug such as cortisone. Once the elbow has healed, no other treatment is necessary. The condition seldom has any long-term effects.

WARNING

MEDICATIONS

Take the following precautions with medications:

- If you are allergic to aspirin or if you have a history of peptic ulcers, you should not take ibuprofen, naproxen, or ketoprofen; ask your doctor about this.
- Do not drink alcohol if you are taking aspirin, acetaminophen, ibuprofen, naproxen, or ketoprofen; combining these painkillers with alcohol increases the risk of liver damage or stomach bleeding.
- If you are pregnant or nursing, talk to your doctor before taking any medication, even one sold over the counter.
- Never give aspirin to a child under 18 years because the drug is linked to a life-threatening condition called Reye's syndrome in children.

How to Prevent Recurring Injury Use elbow pads when you participate in sports. If the injury frequently recurs or if it becomes chronic, your physician may recommend surgically removing the bursa.

GOLFER'S ELBOW

Golfer's elbow is inflammation or a tiny tear in the tendon that attaches the flexor muscle group to the medial epicondyle (inner "knob"). The flexor muscles run down the inside of the forearm and help flex the wrist and close the fingers.

Golfer's elbow, which occurs in both tennis players and golfers, is usually associated with a repetitive motion over time. It can develop from an improper downward stroke in golf, hitting the ground during the golf swing, or improperly executing the forehand stroke in tennis. The condition can also result from underdeveloped flexor muscles. Other sports that can cause golfer's elbow include racquetball, table tennis, rowing, bowling, archery, waterskiing, and weight lifting. Construction work and other kinds of physical activities, such as housework, moving furniture, painting, and gardening, can also cause golfer's elbow.

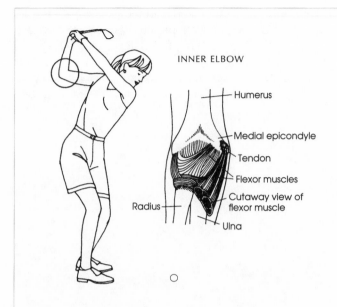

INNER ELBOW

Humerus

Medial epicondyle

Tendon

Flexor muscles

Cutaway view of flexor muscle

Radius

Ulna

GOLFER'S ELBOW

Golfer's elbow is inflammation of the tendon that attaches the flexor muscles to the inner "knob" of the elbow (the medial epicondyle). The condition, also called tendinitis of the elbow, can result from a repetitive motion such as an incorrect downward swing in golf.

SYMPTOMS

Symptoms of golfer's elbow include pain on the inside of the elbow, which can be intense and limit movement. For example, you might feel pain when picking up a child, carrying a heavy tray, or lifting a heavy box.

Immediate Treatment *In serious cases of golfer's elbow (such as if you can't bend or straighten the elbow without pain or you feel numbness or weakness in your arm or hand), see your physician to determine proper treatment.*

Stop the activity that is causing the pain. Place an ice pack on the elbow intermittently (20 minutes every hour while you're awake) for the first 24 to 48 hours after the pain began. Cold treatments help stop internal bleeding and the accumulation of fluids in and around the injured area, thereby decreasing swelling.

SPORTS FIRST AID

283

Unless your doctor has prescribed another medication, take aspirin, ibuprofen, naproxen, or ketoprofen as directed to relieve pain and inflammation. (Acetaminophen relieves pain but has no effect against inflammation; ask your doctor or pharmacist for guidance.) For severe inflammation or for a recurring case, your doctor may recommend an injection of a corticosteroid drug such as cortisone.

WARNING

MEDICATIONS

Take the following precautions with medications:

- If you are allergic to aspirin or if you have a history of peptic ulcers, you should not take ibuprofen, naproxen, or ketoprofen; ask your doctor about this.
- Do not drink alcohol if you are taking aspirin, acetaminophen, ibuprofen, naproxen, or ketoprofen; combining these painkillers with alcohol increases the risk of liver damage or stomach bleeding.
- If you are pregnant or nursing, talk to your doctor before taking any medication, even one sold over the counter.
- Never give aspirin to a child under 18 years because the drug is linked to a life-threatening condition called Reye's syndrome in children.

Continued Care Rest the arm for 4 to 8 weeks. Use an ice pack at least once a day for 2 to 4 days after stopping the activity to reduce swelling and inflammation. Use a heating pad thereafter. Heat increases blood circulation in the area, providing vital nutrients to the injury and helping speed recovery. *Do not* apply heat before the swelling has subsided, or swelling in the injured area may increase. Take aspirin, ibuprofen, naproxen, or ketoprofen as directed to reduce pain and inflammation.

Do not engage in the activity that caused the injury until the pain has subsided. Ease into limited muscle workouts—swing a golf club or tennis racket, lift light weights, and work with a trainer or a physical therapist on hand, wrist, and forearm exercises that strengthen the flexor muscles. Muscle-strengthening exercises also help strengthen the supporting ligaments and tendons. If these measures do not relieve the symptoms, see your physician.

With proper treatment and rest, golfer's elbow seldom has any long-term effects. However, some people experience recurring tendinitis even with preventive measures. In rare cases, surgery to release tension on the tendon, which involves severing the tendon from the bone, may be recommended.

How to Prevent Recurring Injury Allow plenty of time for healing. Use weights and do exercises recommended by a trainer or physical therapist. You may need to continue these measures throughout your life to avoid or reduce pain. Get recommendations from a golf or tennis pro about proper equipment and technique. Your doctor may recommend wearing an elbow brace, which helps constrict the extensor and flexor muscles and helps reduce tension in the areas at which the muscles attach to the elbow. This measure alone can often greatly reduce the pain.

TENNIS ELBOW

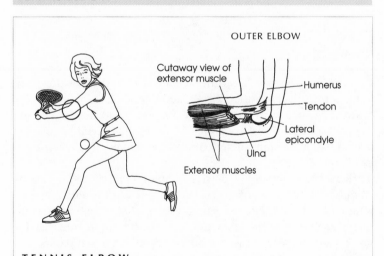

TENNIS ELBOW

Tennis elbow is inflammation of the tendon that attaches the extensor muscles to the outer "knob" of the elbow (the lateral epicondyle). The condition can result from an improperly executed backhand tennis stroke.

Tennis elbow is a catchall phrase for inflammation or a tiny tear in the tendon that connects the extensor muscle group to the lateral epicondyle (the outer "knob"). The extensor muscles—the long muscles on the outside of the forearm—help to extend the wrist.

Tennis elbow, also called elbow tendinitis, is usually associated with a repetitive motion over time. In tennis, it usually develops from an improperly executed backhand stroke. It may also be caused by improper equipment such as a racket that is too stiff or too heavy, a grip that is too small or too large, or strings that are too loose. Other causes include snapping the wrist on a tennis serve or having underdeveloped extensor muscles. Other sports that can cause tennis elbow include racquetball, table tennis, bowling, fly fishing, archery, skiing, and golf. Construction work and other kinds of physical activity such as housework, painting, writing, and gardening can also cause tennis elbow.

SYMPTOMS

The major symptom of tennis elbow is pain on the outside of the elbow, which can be severe and limit movement. Even everyday activities such as shaking hands, holding a coffee cup, turning a doorknob, or picking up a piece of paper may be extremely painful.

Immediate Treatment Stop the activity that is causing the pain. Place an ice pack on the elbow intermittently (20 minutes every hour while you're awake) for the first 24 to 48 hours after the pain began. Cold treatments help stop internal bleeding and the accumulation of fluids in and around the injured area, decreasing swelling.

Unless your doctor has prescribed another medication, take aspirin, ibuprofen, naproxen, or ketoprofen as directed to relieve pain and inflammation. (Acetaminophen relieves pain but has no effect against inflammation; ask your doctor or pharmacist for guidance.) If these measures do not relieve the symptoms, see your physician. He or she may prescribe a different medication to help reduce the pain and swelling. For severe inflammation or for a recurring case, he or she may recommend an injection of a corticosteroid drug such as cortisone.

> ### WARNING
>
> MEDICATIONS
>
> Take the following precautions with medications:
>
> • If you are allergic to aspirin or if you have a history of peptic ulcers, you should not take ibuprofen, naproxen, or ketoprofen; ask your doctor about this.
> • Do not drink alcohol if you are taking aspirin, acetaminophen, ibuprofen, naproxen, or ketoprofen; combining these painkillers with alcohol increases the risk of liver damage or stomach bleeding.
> • If you are pregnant or nursing, talk to your doctor before taking any medication, even one sold over the counter.
> • Never give aspirin to a child under 18 years because the drug is linked to a life-threatening condition called Reye's syndrome in children.

Continued Care Rest the arm for 4 to 8 weeks. Use an ice pack at least once a day for 2 to 4 days after stopping the activity to reduce swelling and inflammation. Use a heating pad thereafter. Heat increases blood circulation in the area, providing vital nutrients to the injury and helping speed recovery. *Do not* apply heat before the swelling has subsided, or swelling in the injured area may increase. Take aspirin, ibuprofen, naproxen, or ketoprofen as directed to reduce the pain and inflammation.

Do not engage in the activity that caused the injury until the pain has subsided. Ease into limited muscle workouts—swing a racket gently, work with light weights, and work with a trainer or a physical therapist on hand, wrist, and forearm exercises that strengthen the extensor muscles. Muscle-strengthening exercises also help strengthen the supporting ligaments and tendons. See your physician if the pain is severe and limits forward motion of the arm.

With proper treatment and rest, tennis elbow seldom has any long-term effects. However, some people experience recurring tendinitis even with precautionary measures. In rare cases,

SPORTS FIRST AID

surgery to release tension on the tendon, which involves severing the tendon from the bone, may be recommended.

How to Prevent Recurring Injury Allow plenty of time for healing. Use weights and do exercises recommended by a trainer or physical therapist. You may need to continue these measures throughout your life to avoid or reduce pain. Get recommendations from a tennis pro about proper equipment and technique. Your doctor may recommend wearing an elbow brace, which helps constrict both the extensor and flexor muscles and helps reduce tension in the areas at which these muscles attach to the elbow. This measure alone can often greatly reduce the pain.

The forefoot or front third of the foot is composed of five singular long bones (metatarsals) that look like the fingers of your hand. The tips of these bones form the toes (phalanges). These bones provide balance for the body.

MORTON'S NEUROMA

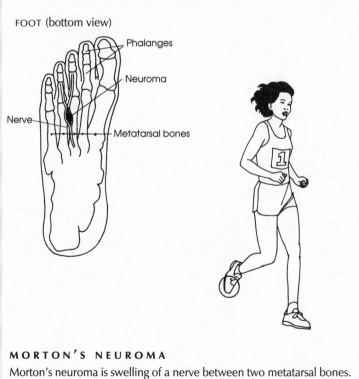

FOOT (bottom view)

Phalanges

Neuroma

Nerve

Metatarsal bones

MORTON'S NEUROMA

Morton's neuroma is swelling of a nerve between two metatarsal bones. Repetitive activities such as running can cause the condition.

Morton's neuroma is pain in the front third of the foot caused by swelling of a nerve between two metatarsal bones, usually those in the third and fourth toes. Poorly fitting shoes and stress on the feet caused by repetitive athletic activity, such as running, are common factors contributing to Morton's neuroma. Genetic susceptibility can also play a part; if the joints of the metatarsal bones are larger than usual, they may compress the nerve between these bones, especially during athletic activity, and cause swelling of the nerve. The condition is common in many sports. Wearing high heels—especially shoes that crowd the toes—may make women more susceptible to this condition.

SYMPTOMS

The major symptoms of Morton's neuroma are pain on the top of the foot, in the ball of the foot, or on the bottom of the toes. The pain may be severe enough to limit athletic participation. Wearing shoes can worsen the pain. In severe cases, the toes may become numb.

Immediate Treatment *If the pain is severe or persistent, if your toes are numb, or if walking causes severe pain, see your physician to determine proper treatment.*

Stop the activity that is causing the pain. Remove your shoes and walk barefoot or in stocking feet. Place an ice pack on the site of the pain intermittently (20 minutes every hour while you're awake) for the first 24 to 48 hours after the injury. Cold treatments help stop internal bleeding and the accumulation of fluid in and around the injured area, thereby decreasing swelling. Elevate your foot above the level of your heart.

Unless your doctor has prescribed another medication, take aspirin, ibuprofen, naproxen, or ketoprofen as directed to relieve pain and inflammation. (Acetaminophen relieves pain but has no effect against inflammation; ask your doctor or pharmacist for guidance.) For severe inflammation or for a recurring case, your doctor may recommend an injection of a corticosteroid drug such as cortisone.

> **WARNING**
>
> MEDICATIONS
>
> Take the following precautions with medications:
>
> - If you are allergic to aspirin or if you have a history of peptic ulcers, you should not take ibuprofen, naproxen, or ketoprofen; ask your doctor about this.
> - Do not drink alcohol if you are taking aspirin, acetaminophen, ibuprofen, naproxen, or ketoprofen; combining these painkillers with alcohol increases the risk of liver damage or stomach bleeding.
> - If you are pregnant or nursing, talk to your doctor before taking any medication, even one sold over the counter.
> - Never give aspirin to a child under 18 years because the drug is linked to a life-threatening condition called Reye's syndrome in children.

Continued Care Rest the foot for 3 to 6 weeks. Do not engage in the activity that caused the neuroma until the pain has subsided. Use an ice pack to reduce any swelling that may occur. Take aspirin, ibuprofen, naproxen, or ketoprofen to relieve pain and inflammation. See your physician if the pain in your foot or the numbness in your toes continues. With proper treatment and rest, Morton's neuroma seldom has any long-term effects.

How to Prevent Recurring Injury The most important preventive measure is to wear shoes that give your foot room to move.

PLANTAR FASCIITIS

Plantar fasciitis, or heel spur, is a common injury to the plantar fascia, a band of protective tissue that runs from the heel along the bottom of the foot to the base of the toes. In plantar fasciitis, the plantar fascia detaches slightly from the heel, causing pain and inflammation in the bottom of the heel that hurts more when standing on the toes. The injury can range from a tiny tear to a more serious, but rare, severing of the plantar fascia. Regardless of the extent of the tear, a spokelike calcium deposit, or "spur," can form at the heel bone, aggravating the condition.

Plantar fasciitis is usually caused by overuse, as in frequent running. It also can result from poor arches, from wearing shoes with a stiff heel, or from running or competing in sports on hard terrain, such as concrete. The condition can also result from an increase in body weight. Other sports in which the injury can occur include aerobics, baseball, basketball, football, hiking, rugby, soccer, tennis, and track and field. Women who regularly wear high heels and do not stretch their calf muscles and the plantar fascia before engaging in sports may be susceptible to this injury.

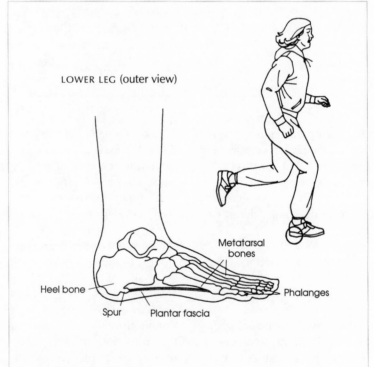

LOWER LEG (outer view)

Metatarsal bones

Heel bone

Phalanges

Spur

Plantar fascia

PLANTAR FASCIITIS

Plantar fasciitis, or heel spur, is a tear in the plantar fascia that is aggravated by a spur that develops at the heel bone. The injury often results from repetitive motion such as running.

SYMPTOMS

The major symptom of plantar fasciitis is pain in the heel, especially when waking. Ironically, walking may hurt, but running, once the feet and legs have been warmed up, does not. The pain usually subsides when you are lying down but may return when you get up. Your heel may be swollen and bruised. You may feel as though you are walking on a pea or pebble.

Immediate Treatment *If you are unable to place any pressure on your foot, or if walking or climbing stairs causes intense pain, see your physician to determine proper treatment.*

Stop the activity that is causing the pain. Place an ice pack on the heel intermittently (20 minutes every hour while you're awake) for the first 24 to 48 hours after the injury. Cold treatments help stop internal bleeding and the accumulation of fluids in and around the injured area, thereby decreasing swelling. Elevate your foot above the level of your heart. Unless your doctor has prescribed another medication, take aspirin, ibuprofen, naproxen, or ketoprofen as directed to relieve pain and inflammation. (Acetaminophen relieves pain but has no effect against inflammation; ask your doctor or pharmacist for guidance.)

WARNING

MEDICATIONS

Take the following precautions with medications:

- If you are allergic to aspirin or if you have a history of peptic ulcers, you should not take ibuprofen, naproxen, or ketoprofen; ask your doctor about this.
- Do not drink alcohol if you are taking aspirin, acetaminophen, ibuprofen, naproxen, or ketoprofen; combining these painkillers with alcohol increases the risk of liver damage or stomach bleeding.
- If you are pregnant or nursing, talk to your doctor before taking any medication, even one sold over the counter.
- Never give aspirin to a child under 18 years because the drug is linked to a life-threatening condition called Reye's syndrome in children.

SPORTS FIRST AID

Continued Care Keep your legs slightly elevated and extended straight out in front of you and stay off your feet as much as possible for 3 to 6 weeks. Do not engage in the activity that caused the injury until the pain has subsided. With your physician's okay, work with a trainer or physical therapist on exercises that stretch the plantar fascia. Take aspirin, ibuprofen, naproxen, or ketoprofen as directed to relieve pain and inflammation. If the pain and swelling continue, see your physician. In rare cases, surgery to release tension on the fascia, which involves severing the fascia from the heel bone, may be recommended.

How to Prevent Recurring Injury Allow plenty of time for the injury to heal before resuming your activity. Your physician, trainer, or physical therapist may recommend using shoe inserts when you engage in sports to help relieve pressure on the heel. Carefully perform exercises that stretch the calf muscles and the plantar fascia; always do these exercises to warm up before engaging in sports. Wear proper shoes. A stiff heel in running shoes or tennis shoes can cause or aggravate the condition. Run or train on a dirt or wood track, not on concrete.

STRESS FRACTURE IN THE FOOT

A stress fracture usually occurs in the foot or in the tibia (one of the lower leg bones). A stress fracture in the foot is a hairline crack in one of the metatarsal bones. The injury can result from a repetitive motion, such as running, from sudden stress placed on the foot, such as a change in running routine or running surface, or from participating in sports after a period of inactivity. It also can result from an increase in body weight. Stress fractures are common in many sports other than running, including gymnastics, aerobics, baseball, basketball, tennis, rugby, soccer, and walking. Any activity that puts stress on the feet or legs over time may cause a stress fracture.

SYMPTOMS

A stress fracture causes intense pain at the site of the fracture. During exercise, the foot or leg may feel like it is on fire. The pain subsides when you stop the activity. In more serious cases, the pain may continue even after stopping the activity.

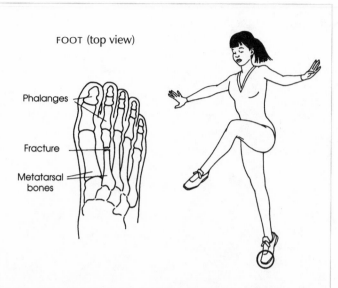

FOOT (top view)

Phalanges

Fracture

Metatarsal
bones

STRESS FRACTURE IN THE FOOT
A stress fracture usually occurs in the foot or in the tibia, one of the lower leg bones. A stress fracture in the foot is a hairline crack in one of the metatarsal bones, which can occur when all the weight of the body is put on these bones.

Immediate Treatment *If the pain is severe and persistent, see your physician to determine proper treatment.*

Stop the activity that is causing the pain. Place an ice pack on the area intermittently (20 minutes every hour while you're awake) for the first 24 to 48 hours after the injury. Cold treatments help stop internal bleeding and the accumulation of fluids in and around the injured area, thereby decreasing swelling. Elevate your foot above the level of your heart. Unless your doctor has prescribed another medication, take aspirin, ibuprofen, naproxen, or ketoprofen as directed to relieve pain and inflammation. (Acetaminophen relieves pain but has no effect against inflammation; ask your doctor or pharmacist for guidance.)

> ### WARNING
>
> MEDICATIONS
>
> Take the following precautions with medications:
>
> • If you are allergic to aspirin or if you have a history of peptic ulcers, you should not take ibuprofen, naproxen, or ketoprofen; ask your doctor about this.
> • Do not drink alcohol if you are taking aspirin, acetaminophen, ibuprofen, naproxen, or ketoprofen; combining these painkillers with alcohol increases the risk of liver damage or stomach bleeding.
> • If you are pregnant or nursing, talk to your doctor before taking any medication, even one sold over the counter.
> • Never give aspirin to a child under 18 years because the drug is linked to a life-threatening condition called Reye's syndrome in children.

Continued Care Rest the foot for 4 to 6 weeks. Do not engage in the activity that caused the injury until the pain has subsided. Use an ice pack at the site of the injury at least once a day to help reduce the pain and inflammation. Take aspirin, ibuprofen, naproxen, or ketoprofen as directed to reduce pain and inflammation. See your physician if the pain continues after you resume activity. With proper treatment and rest, stress fractures seldom have any long-term effects.

How to Prevent Recurring Injury Resume activity gradually, especially sports that involve running. Wear proper shoes. Run or train on a soft surface, such as a dirt or wood track, not concrete. Increase your speed or distance gradually.

The hand consists of the bones and joints of the fingers and thumb (called phalanges), the five metacarpal bones of the palm, and eight small, oblong bones that together form the wrist. Beneath the skin is a complex network of ligaments, tendons, and muscles. Muscles in the forearm allow the hand to perform a wide range of motion and tasks.

BASEBALL FINGER

Baseball finger is a tear in a tendon at the joint at the end of the finger. Depending on the severity of the injury, you may not be able to straighten the finger. The injury is caused by sudden force exerted on the end of the finger, such as from a thrown or hit baseball.

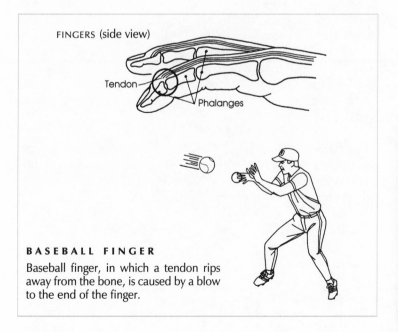

FINGERS (side view)

Tendon

Phalanges

BASEBALL FINGER
Baseball finger, in which a tendon rips away from the bone, is caused by a blow to the end of the finger.

SYMPTOMS

Baseball finger causes immediate pain, swelling, and bruising at the site of the injury.

Immediate Treatment Place an ice pack on the finger intermittently (20 minutes every hour while you're awake) for the first 24 to 48 hours after the injury. Cold treatments help stop internal bleeding and the accumulation of fluids in and around the injured area, thereby decreasing swelling. Elevate your finger above the level of your heart. See your physician to determine the extent of the injury. Your physician may recommend using a splint on the finger to aid healing.

Unless your doctor has prescribed another medication, take aspirin, ibuprofen, naproxen, or ketoprofen as directed to relieve pain and inflammation. (Acetaminophen relieves pain but has no effect against inflammation; ask your doctor or pharmacist for guidance.)

WARNING

MEDICATIONS

Take the following precautions with medications:

- If you are allergic to aspirin or if you have a history of peptic ulcers, you should not take ibuprofen, naproxen, or ketoprofen; ask your doctor about this.
- Do not drink alcohol if you are taking aspirin, acetaminophen, ibuprofen, naproxen, or ketoprofen; combining these painkillers with alcohol increases the risk of liver damage or stomach bleeding.
- If you are pregnant or nursing, talk to your doctor before taking any medication, even one sold over the counter.
- Never give aspirin to a child under 18 years because the drug is linked to a life-threatening condition called Reye's syndrome in children.

Continued Care Do not engage in the activity that caused the injury until the pain has subsided. Work with a trainer or physical therapist on exercises that strengthen the tendons in the fingers. Use an ice pack to reduce any swelling that may occur. Take aspirin, ibuprofen, naproxen, or ketoprofen as directed to relieve pain and inflammation. See your physician if the pain continues or injury recurs. With proper treatment and rest, this injury seldom has any long-term effects, although it sometimes results in the permanent inability to completely straighten the end joint of the finger. This lack of movement seldom interferes in any way with the functioning of the finger, but you should still see your physician if you cannot straighten the end joint of the injured finger.

How to Prevent Recurring Injury Continue doing exercises that strengthen the tendons in the finger. Use good judgment when engaging in your sport.

SKIER'S THUMB

Skier's thumb is a tear or complete severing of the ligament that attaches the thumb to one of the metacarpal bones in the palm. The injury often occurs during a fall in skiing when the ski pole forces the thumb away from the fingers. It can also occur when catching a swiftly thrown baseball, football, or basketball.

SYMPTOMS

Skier's thumb causes immediate pain and swelling at the base of the thumb. The pain may intensify and bruising may occur several hours after the injury. Pinching may be difficult.

Immediate Treatment Place an ice pack on the base of the thumb intermittently (20 minutes every hour while you're awake) for the first 24 to 48 hours after the injury. Cold treatments help stop internal bleeding and the accumulation of fluids in and around the injured area, thereby decreasing swelling. Elevate your hand above the level of your heart. See your physician to determine the extent of the injury. Your physician may recommend using a splint on the thumb to aid healing.

SPORTS FIRST AID

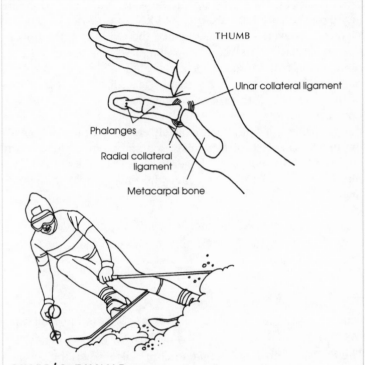

THUMB

Ulnar collateral ligament

Phalanges

Radial collateral ligament

Metacarpal bone

SKIER'S THUMB

Skier's thumb is a tear or a complete severing of the ligament that attaches the thumb to the metacarpal bone. The injury often occurs during a skiing fall when the ski pole forces the thumb away from the fingers.

Unless your doctor has prescribed another medication, take aspirin, ibuprofen, naproxen, or ketoprofen as directed to relieve pain and inflammation. (Acetaminophen relieves pain but has no effect against inflammation; ask your doctor or pharmacist for guidance.)

MEDICATIONS

Take the following precautions with medications:

- If you are allergic to aspirin or if you have a history of peptic ulcers, you should not take ibuprofen, naproxen, or ketoprofen; ask your doctor about this.
- Do not drink alcohol if you are taking aspirin, acetaminophen, ibuprofen, naproxen, or ketoprofen; combining these painkillers with alcohol increases the risk of liver damage or stomach bleeding.
- If you are pregnant or nursing, talk to your doctor before taking any medication, even one sold over the counter.
- Never give aspirin to a child under 18 years because the drug is linked to a life-threatening condition called Reye's syndrome in children.

Continued Care Do not engage in the activity that caused the injury until the pain has subsided. Work with a trainer or physical therapist on exercises that strengthen the tendons and ligaments in the hand. Use an ice pack when necessary to reduce swelling. Take aspirin, ibuprofen, naproxen, or ketoprofen as directed to relieve pain and inflammation. If the pain continues or if the injury recurs, see your physician.

With proper treatment and rest, the injury seldom has long-term effects. In serious cases, surgery will be necessary to repair the ligament.

How to Prevent Recurring Injury Continue doing exercises that strengthen the tendons and ligaments in the hand. Use good judgment when engaging in your sport.

The hip consists of the ilium bone (the top of the pelvis), the sacrum and coccyx (tailbone) of the lower spine, the pubic bone, and the ischium bone (the bottom of the pelvis). Several muscle-tendon groups are connected to the hip. The bones of the hip protect the internal organs and allow standing and movement.

HIP POINTER

A hip pointer is a bruise or tear in a muscle that attaches to the top of the ilium bone at the waist. The injury, which is very common in contact sports, is caused by a blow to or fall on the hip.

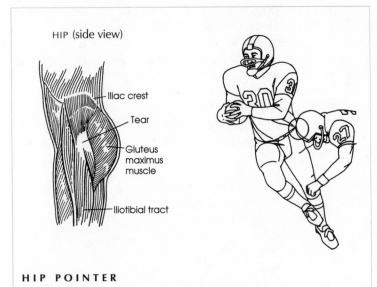

HIP (side view)

Iliac crest

Tear

Gluteus maximus muscle

Iliotibial tract

HIP POINTER

A hip pointer is a bruise or tear in a muscle that attaches to the top of the ilium bone at the waist. The injury results from a blow to or fall on the hip.

SYMPTOMS

A hip pointer causes pain and bruising in the hip. The pain may intensify several hours after the injury.

Immediate Treatment *If the pain is severe or persistent, see your physician to determine proper treatment.*

Place an ice pack on the hip intermittently (20 minutes every hour while you're awake) for the first 24 to 48 hours after the injury. Cold treatments help stop internal bleeding and the accumulation of fluids in and around the injured area, thereby decreasing swelling.

Unless your doctor has prescribed another medication, take aspirin, ibuprofen, naproxen, or ketoprofen as directed to relieve pain and inflammation. (Acetaminophen relieves pain but has no effect against inflammation; ask your doctor or pharmacist for guidance.)

WARNING

MEDICATIONS

Take the following precautions with medications:

- If you are allergic to aspirin or if you have a history of peptic ulcers, you should not take ibuprofen, naproxen, or ketoprofen; ask your doctor about this.
- Do not drink alcohol if you are taking aspirin, acetaminophen, ibuprofen, naproxen, or ketoprofen; combining these painkillers with alcohol increases the risk of liver damage or stomach bleeding.
- If you are pregnant or nursing, talk to your doctor before taking any medication, even one sold over the counter.
- Never give aspirin to a child under 18 years because the drug is linked to a life-threatening condition called Reye's syndrome in children.

SPORTS FIRST AID

Continued Care Use an ice pack at least once a day for 2 to 4 days after the injury. Take aspirin, ibuprofen, naproxen, or ketoprofen as directed to relieve the pain and inflammation. After the swelling has stopped, place a heating pad on the hip at least once a day until the injury heals. Heat increases blood circulation in the area, providing vital nutrients to the injury and helping speed recovery. *Do not* apply heat before the swelling has subsided, or swelling in the injured area may increase. Avoid athletic activity until the injury has had time to heal, or until the pain in the hip has gone. The length of time for the injury to heal depends on the severity of the tear and can range from 3 to 6 weeks or longer.

After the injury has healed, gradually and carefully perform exercises that involve stretching the muscles in your upper legs and waist. Use an ice pack to reduce swelling when necessary. See your physician if the pain continues or if the injury recurs. With proper rest, hip pointers seldom have any long-term effects.

How to Prevent Recurring Injury Wear hip padding when you engage in contact sports.

KNEE

The knee consists of three main bones—the femur of the upper leg, and the tibia and fibula of the lower leg. These bones are connected by a series of ligaments to form the knee joint. Resting on top of the knee joint is a fourth bone, the patella (kneecap). Bursas (fluid-filled sacs or saclike cavities) surround and cushion the bones. Muscles, such as the quadriceps in the front upper leg and the hamstrings in the back upper leg, are connected to these bones by tendons. Muscles, tendons, and ligaments add stability to the joint. The knee, like the elbow, is a hinge joint that allows the leg to extend and bend.

RUNNER'S KNEE

Runner's knee, or patellofemoral joint pain, is a common problem that affects runners and other athletes of all abilities. The term refers to damage to and roughness of the cartilage that covers the undersurface of the kneecap. Cartilage covers all bone and joint surfaces and acts as a shock absorber to keep bone from rubbing against bone. When the condition occurs, rough spots on the kneecap can rub directly against the femur, causing pain.

Runner's knee can result from a repetitive motion (such as running) or sudden stress on the knee (which can result from a change in running routine or running surface, using heavier weights in weight lifting, or using a high gear in bicycling). It also may be influenced by genetic factors (a "loose" kneecap or an abnormality in the structure of the kneecap), by a direct or forceful blow to the kneecap, or by unknown factors. Any sport in which pressure is put on the knees—such as weight lifting, football, tennis, rowing, aerobics, or bicycling—can cause runner's knee. Other activities that can cause runner's knee include heavy lifting or stair climbing.

Runner's knee has also been described as pain on the outside

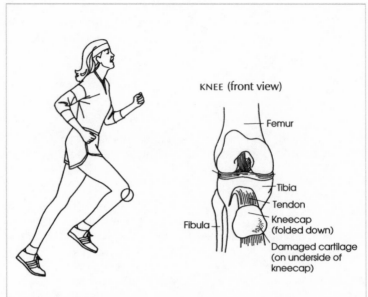

KNEE (front view)

Femur

Tibia

Tendon

Kneecap
(folded down)

Fibula

Damaged cartilage
(on underside of
kneecap)

RUNNER'S KNEE

Runner's knee—pain on or behind the knee—is caused by damage to the cartilage that covers the undersurface of the kneecap. The injury often results from running, which puts repetitive stress on the knee.

of one or both knees. This condition, although not as common as patellofemoral joint pain, is usually caused by overuse—for example, by increasing running mileage without acclimating first to the new distance. The pain in the knee occurs when the foot strikes the ground at a pronounced angle while running, which puts extra stress on, and may cause a tiny tear in a strip of connective tissue that extends from the ilium (hipbone) to the top of the tibia. Usually, the outside of the person's shoe and the heel are worn down. If you have any of these signs and symptoms, see your physician for proper diagnosis and treatment. The condition can be corrected with shoe inserts, moldings that fit inside the shoes to give the feet support and help the feet strike the ground properly during running.

SYMPTOMS

Symptoms of runner's knee include anything from a dull ache to a sharp pain on and behind the kneecap, pain while sitting with the knees bent, pain when kneeling or squatting, or pain when walking up or down stairs. The condition can also cause swelling of the knee, muscle weakness in the quadriceps, or grinding and popping of the knee.

Immediate Treatment *If the pain is persistent or severe or if your knee is swollen, see your physician to determine proper treatment.*

Stop the activity that is causing the pain. Place an ice pack on the knee intermittently (20 minutes every hour while you're awake) for the first 24 to 48 hours after the injury. Cold treatments help stop internal bleeding and the accumulation of fluids in and around the injured area, thereby decreasing swelling. Keep your leg elevated above the level of your heart.

Unless your doctor has prescribed another medication, take aspirin, ibuprofen, naproxen, or ketoprofen as directed to relieve pain and inflammation. (Acetaminophen relieves pain but has no effect against inflammation; ask your doctor or pharmacist for guidance.)

WARNING

MEDICATIONS

Take the following precautions with medications:

- If you are allergic to aspirin or if you have a history of peptic ulcers, you should not take ibuprofen, naproxen, or ketoprofen; ask your doctor about this.
- Do not drink alcohol if you are taking aspirin, acetaminophen, ibuprofen, naproxen, or ketoprofen; combining these painkillers with alcohol increases the risk of liver damage or stomach bleeding.
- If you are pregnant or nursing, talk to your doctor before taking any medication, even one sold over the counter.
- Never give aspirin to a child under 18 years because the drug is linked to a life-threatening condition called Reye's syndrome in children.

SPORTS FIRST AID

Continued Care Rest the legs for approximately 3 to 6 weeks. Use ice for 2 to 4 days after stopping the activity to reduce swelling and inflammation. Occasional use of an elastic bandage on the knee may help promote stability and prevent further injury. If you have peripheral vascular disease or diabetes, however, you should consult your physician first before using an elastic bandage. Keep your legs slightly elevated.

Do not engage in the activity that caused the injury until the pain has subsided. With your physician's okay, work with a trainer or physical therapist on exercises that strengthen the quadriceps muscles. Use an ice pack to reduce any swelling that may occur. Take aspirin, ibuprofen, naproxen, or ketoprofen as directed to relieve pain and inflammation. If the pain and swelling continue, see your physician.

Long-Term Effects Some pain may continue when the knee is bent. You may have difficulty kneeling or squatting. In some cases, surgery may be recommended to smooth the roughness on the back of the kneecap.

How to Prevent Recurring Injury Keep your quadriceps muscles strong with muscle-strengthening exercises that also help strengthen the joint-supporting ligaments and tendons. Use good judgment in increasing your running mileage and intensity or when running on a different surface. Don't use the high gears when bicycling. Gradually acclimate yourself to lifting heavy objects. Ensure that your shoes fit properly.

TORN CARTILAGE IN THE KNEE

Meniscus cartilage is a crescent-shaped band of elastic tissue inside joints. The knee joint has two menisci that sit on top of the tibia, the large lower leg bone. The lateral meniscus is on the inner side of the joint and the medial meniscus is on the outer side. This cartilage helps the knee joint fit snugly together and helps distribute body weight evenly over the surface of the tibia. Injury to the meniscus cartilage can range from a tiny tear to a complete rupture, which, in most cases, must be repaired surgically. What may begin as a small tear can, with repeated twists or blows to the knee, develop into a complete severing.

The injury is usually caused by a severe twist or forceful blow

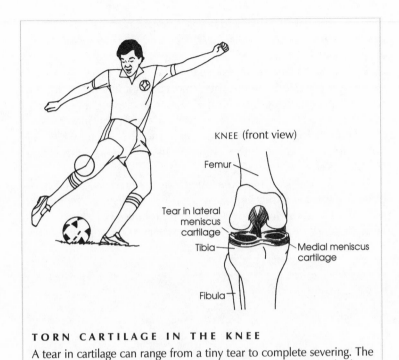

KNEE (front view)

Femur

Tear in lateral
meniscus
cartilage

Tibia

Medial meniscus
cartilage

Fibula

TORN CARTILAGE IN THE KNEE

A tear in cartilage can range from a tiny tear to complete severing. The injury is usually caused by a severe twist or forceful blow to the knee when the leg is straightened.

to the knee when the leg is straightened. It also can result from force placed on the knee when the foot is planted while the leg is straightened, causing the knee to twist. Torn cartilage sometimes occurs in conjunction with a torn ligament in the knee. The injury is very common in contact sports such as football. Other sports in which the injury can occur include hockey, lacrosse, soccer, downhill skiing, basketball, and golf. Torn cartilage in the knee can also result from tripping over objects or falling with force on the knee.

SYMPTOMS

The major symptom of torn cartilage in the knee is pain at the joint line (the area at which the bones of the leg join to form the knee). The knee may lock or buckle, make a popping sound, or swell.

Immediate Treatment *See a physician for proper diagnosis of the extent of the tear. Surgery may be recommended to repair or remove the damaged cartilage.*

Stop the activity that is causing the pain. (The pain and swelling are likely to keep you from continuing.) Apply an ice pack to the knee intermittently (20 minutes every hour while you're awake) for the first 24 to 48 hours after the injury. Cold treatments help stop internal bleeding and the accumulation of fluids in and around the injured area, thereby decreasing swelling. Keep your leg slightly elevated.

Unless your doctor has prescribed another medication, take aspirin, ibuprofen, naproxen, or ketoprofen as directed to relieve pain and inflammation. (Acetaminophen relieves pain but has no effect against inflammation; ask your doctor or pharmacist for guidance.)

WARNING

MEDICATIONS

Take the following precautions with medications:

- If you are allergic to aspirin or if you have a history of peptic ulcers, you should not take ibuprofen, naproxen, or ketoprofen; ask your doctor about this.
- Do not drink alcohol if you are taking aspirin, acetaminophen, ibuprofen, naproxen, or ketoprofen; combining these painkillers with alcohol increases the risk of liver damage or stomach bleeding.
- If you are pregnant or nursing, talk to your doctor before taking any medication, even one sold over the counter.
- Never give aspirin to a child under 18 years because the drug is linked to a life-threatening condition called Reye's syndrome in children.

Continued Care Follow your physician's instructions regarding follow-up care. See your physician if the pain and swelling continue or if your knee locks or buckles.

Long-Term Effects You may have some stiffness and swelling in your knee. The injury may make you susceptible to developing arthritis or ligament tears in your knee.

How to Prevent Recurring Injury With your physician's okay, work with a trainer or physical therapist to strengthen the hamstring muscles in your back upper leg and the quadriceps muscles in the front upper leg.

TORN LIGAMENT

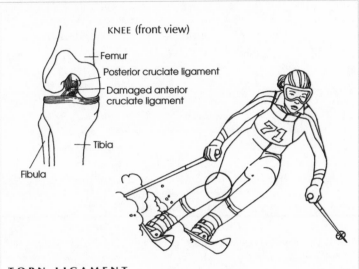

KNEE (front view)

Femur

Posterior cruciate ligament

Damaged anterior cruciate ligament

Tibia

Fibula

TORN LIGAMENT

Damage to the anterior cruciate ligament, which provides stability to the knee joint, is a common injury in sports. It often occurs when extra force is placed on the knee when the foot is planted while the leg is straightened.

Damage to the anterior cruciate ligament—often referred to as an ACL injury—is one of the most common injuries in sports, after sprained ankles. The anterior cruciate ligament is one of two ligaments that crisscross inside the knee and add stability to the joint. An injury can range from a tiny tear to a complete rupture of the ligament. A tear in the ligament may be accompanied by torn cartilage in the knee.

SPORTS FIRST AID

311

The injury is caused by a traumatic or sudden blow to the knee when the leg is straightened. It also can occur from force placed on the knee when the foot is planted while the leg is straightened. The injury is very common in contact sports such as football. Other sports in which the injury can occur include lacrosse, soccer, downhill skiing, and basketball. The injury can also result from tripping over an object on the floor.

SYMPTOMS

A torn ligament in the knee can cause swelling and pain from the accumulation of fluid and blood inside the joint. The injury can also cause stiffness, limitation of movement, or displacement of the knee. You may hear a popping sound when the ligament is torn. Depending on the severity of the tear, the symptoms may not appear for 6 to 12 hours.

Immediate Treatment *If the pain is severe or persistent, if your knee is swollen, or if the movement in your knee is limited, see your physician to determine proper treatment. Depending on the severity of the injury, he or she may recommend surgery to reconstruct the ligament.*

Stop the activity that is causing the pain. Apply an ice pack to the knee intermittently (20 minutes every hour while you're awake) for the first 24 to 48 hours after the injury. Cold treatments help stop internal bleeding and the accumulation of fluids in and around the injured area, thereby decreasing swelling. Keep your leg slightly elevated.

Unless your doctor has prescribed another medication, take aspirin, ibuprofen, naproxen, or ketoprofen as directed to relieve pain and inflammation. (Acetaminophen relieves pain but has no effect against inflammation; ask your doctor or pharmacist for guidance.)

> **WARNING**
>
> MEDICATIONS
>
> Take the following precautions with medications:
>
> - If you are allergic to aspirin or if you have a history of peptic ulcers, you should not take ibuprofen, naproxen, or ketoprofen; ask your doctor about this.
> - Do not drink alcohol if you are taking aspirin, acetaminophen, ibuprofen, naproxen, or ketoprofen; combining these painkillers with alcohol increases the risk of liver damage or stomach bleeding.
> - If you are pregnant or nursing, talk to your doctor before taking any medication, even one sold over the counter.
> - Never give aspirin to a child under 18 years because the drug is linked to a life-threatening condition called Reye's syndrome in children.

Continued Care Follow your physician's instructions regarding follow-up care. See your physician if the pain or swelling in your knee continues or if your knee buckles.

Long-Term Effects The knee may be unstable and give out, especially when you turn sharply to the left or right, such as when cutting in football. Your knee may be susceptible to cartilage tears because it is looser than normal. Your knee may also be susceptible to arthritic changes over time.

How to Prevent Recurring Injury With your physician's okay, work with a trainer or physical therapist to strengthen the leg muscles, especially the hamstring muscles in the back upper leg. Muscle-strengthening exercises also help strengthen the joint-supporting ligaments and tendons.

SPORTS FIRST AID

313

ACHILLES TENDINITIS

Achilles tendinitis is a tear in the tendon that attaches the calf muscles to the heel bone. Injury to the Achilles tendon can range from a tiny tear to a more serious rupture of the tendon. The Achilles tendon, one of the longest and strongest tendons in the body, allows you to run, climb, and stand on the tips of your toes.

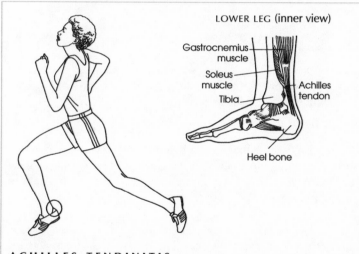

LOWER LEG (inner view)

Gastrocnemius muscle

Soleus muscle

Tibia

Achilles tendon

Heel bone

ACHILLES TENDINITIS

Achilles tendinitis is a strain or tear in the tendon that attaches the calf muscles to the heel bone. The injury frequently results from a repetitive movement such as running.

Achilles tendinitis can result from repetitive motion such as running over time, or from sudden stress placed on the tendon, such as in sprinting. A tear can also occur if the tendon is fatigued from overuse or if pressure is placed on it before a sufficient warm-up period, from wearing improper shoes during sports activities or athletic shoes with a stiff heel, or from running or training on a hard surface. The injury can occur in any sport, but is most common in aerobics, baseball, basketball, football, hiking, rugby, soccer, tennis, and track and field. The injury can also result from everyday activities such as running for a bus or taking long walks without acclimating first to the distance.

SYMPTOMS

Depending on the extent of the tear, symptoms can range from mild discomfort to severe pain that may be centered at the lower back of the leg (about 2 inches above the ankle). With a mild strain or tear, the pain may be noticeable on waking up in the morning, but, as the tendon warms up during walking or exercise, the pain may disappear. However, the discomfort may return the next morning. With a more serious tear or severing of the tendon, you may feel as if someone kicked you in the back of the leg as the tendon ruptures. With both minor and major injuries to the tendon, pain and swelling (from the accumulation of fluids) will worsen several hours after the onset of the injury.

Immediate Treatment *If the pain is severe or persistent, see your physician to determine proper treatment. A complete rupture usually has to be repaired surgically.*

Stop the activity that caused the injury. Apply an ice pack to the area intermittently (20 minutes every hour while you're awake) for the first 24 to 48 hours after the injury. Cold treatments help stop internal bleeding and the accumulation of fluids in and around the injured area, thereby decreasing swelling. Keep your leg slightly elevated.

Unless your doctor has prescribed another medication, take aspirin, ibuprofen, naproxen, or ketoprofen as directed to relieve pain and inflammation. (Acetaminophen relieves pain but has no effect against inflammation; ask your doctor or pharmacist for guidance.)

WARNING

MEDICATIONS

Take the following precautions with medications:

- If you are allergic to aspirin or if you have a history of peptic ulcers, you should not take ibuprofen, naproxen, or ketoprofen; ask your doctor about this.
- Do not drink alcohol if you are taking aspirin, acetaminophen, ibuprofen, naproxen, or ketoprofen; combining these painkillers with alcohol increases the risk of liver damage or stomach bleeding.
- If you are pregnant or nursing, talk to your doctor before taking any medication, even one sold over the counter.
- Never give aspirin to a child under 18 years because the drug is linked to a life-threatening condition called Reye's syndrome in children.

Continued Care Do not engage in the activity that caused the injury until the pain has subsided. Gradually and carefully extend or stretch your lower leg and foot. Work with a trainer or physical therapist on light exercises that stretch the calf muscles and the Achilles tendon. He or she may recommend that you wear half-inch lifts in your shoes to take pressure off the heel. Use an ice pack to reduce any swelling that may occur. Take aspirin, ibuprofen, naproxen, or ketoprofen as directed to relieve pain and inflammation. See your physician if the pain and swelling persist.

With proper treatment and rest, Achilles tendinitis seldom has any long-term effects. However, some people experience recurring tendinitis regardless of preventive measures. In rare cases, surgery may be recommended to remove scar tissue and part of the tendon.

How to Prevent Recurring Injury Allow plenty of time for the injury to heal. Your physician, trainer, or physical therapist may recommend that you wear shoe inserts when you engage in sports to help relieve pressure on your heel. Carefully perform exercises that stretch the calf muscles and the Achilles tendon. Wear proper shoes—a stiff heel in running shoes or tennis shoes can cause or aggravate the condition. Run or train on a dirt or wood track (not on concrete).

CALF MUSCLE TEAR

Injury to the calf muscle can range from a tiny tear to a complete rupture. A tear in the calf muscle usually occurs in people who participate in sports after a period of inactivity. The injury usually occurs when they jump and land on their toes. The calf muscles, the gastrocnemius and the soleus, extend from the back of the knee to the heel. The gastrocnemius muscle starts behind the knee and forms the bulky part of the calf. The soleus muscle starts lower down at the back of the shin. The two muscles join to form the Achilles tendon, which connects them to the heel. The calf muscles pull the heel up to allow a springing movement through the toes, which is important for walking, running, jumping, and hopping.

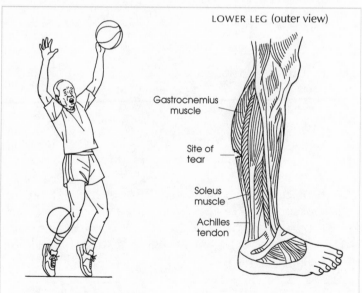

LOWER LEG (outer view)

Gastrocnemius muscle

Site of tear

Soleus muscle

Achilles tendon

CALF MUSCLE TEAR

A tear in a calf muscle usually results from jumping and landing on the toes. The injury is most common in people who are not used to athletic activity.

SYMPTOMS

Symptoms of a torn calf muscle include an immediate sharp pain in the middle of the calf, sometimes accompanied by a snapping or tearing sensation. The middle of the calf muscle may swell and feel tender to the touch.

Immediate Treatment *If your calf swells, if the pain is not relieved by lifting your heel, or if you cannot walk, see your physician to determine treatment.*

Elevate your heel by wearing a heel lift in your shoe to take pressure off the calf muscle. Unless your doctor has prescribed another medication, take aspirin, ibuprofen, naproxen, or keto-profen as directed to relieve pain and inflammation. (Aceta-minophen relieves pain but has no effect against inflammation; ask your doctor or pharmacist for guidance.)

WARNING

MEDICATIONS

Take the following precautions with medications:

- If you are allergic to aspirin or if you have a history of peptic ulcers, you should not take ibuprofen, naproxen, or ketoprofen; ask your doctor about this.
- Do not drink alcohol if you are taking aspirin, acetaminophen, ibuprofen, naproxen, or ketoprofen; combining these painkillers with alcohol increases the risk of liver damage or stomach bleeding.
- If you are pregnant or nursing, talk to your doctor before taking any medication, even one sold over the counter.
- Never give aspirin to a child under 18 years because the drug is linked to a life-threatening condition called Reye's syndrome in children.

Continued Care Once the injury heals, no treatment is necessary. A tear in the calf muscle seldom has any long-term effects.

How to Prevent Recurring Injury Always warm up your calf muscles with a few minutes of stretching exercises before engaging in sports.

HAMSTRING MUSCLE PULL

Injury to the hamstring can range from a tiny tear to a more serious tear in the muscle or in the tendons that attach the muscle to bone. Most injuries occur in the muscle. The hamstring is a large muscle on the back of the thigh that runs from the bottom of the pelvis to the top of the knee. About mid-thigh, the hamstring separates into two major muscle-tendon groups. The medial (inner) hamstring tendons attach to the inner knee and the front of the tibia (one of the lower leg bones). The lateral (outer) hamstring tendons attach to the outside of the knee at the top of the fibula (the other lower leg bone). The hamstring muscle bends the leg. (The quadriceps muscle on the front of the thigh extends or straightens the leg.)

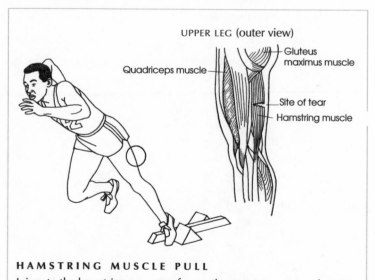

UPPER LEG (outer view)

Gluteus maximus muscle

Quadriceps muscle

Site of tear

Hamstring muscle

HAMSTRING MUSCLE PULL

Injury to the hamstring can range from a tiny tear to a more serious tear in the muscle or in the tendons that attach the muscle to bone. The injury usually occurs during a quick running start, such as a sprint, when the leg is straightened rather than bent at the knee.

SPORTS FIRST AID

319

Injury to the hamstring is common among athletes of all abilities. It usually results from a quick start, such as sprinting when the leg is straightened. The injury can also occur when the quadriceps muscle is overdeveloped in relation to the hamstring muscle or when engaging in sports before a sufficient warm-up period. Some people have naturally tight hamstrings that may or may not make them susceptible to injury. Sports in which a hamstring injury can occur include baseball, football, basketball, rugby, soccer, and tennis.

SYMPTOMS

The major symptom of a hamstring muscle pull is pain in the back of the leg. The degree of pain depends on the severity of the tear. With some tears or strains in the muscle, pain may worsen over several hours, making it difficult to walk, sit, or bend over.

Immediate Treatment *If the pain in the back of the leg is severe or persistent or if you cannot straighten your leg, see your physician to determine proper treatment.*

Stop the activity that is causing the pain. Place an ice pack on the back of the leg intermittently (20 minutes every hour while you're awake) for the first 24 to 48 hours after the injury. Cold treatments help stop internal bleeding and the accumulation of fluids in and around the injured area, thereby decreasing swelling. Keep your leg slightly elevated.

Unless your doctor has prescribed another medication, take aspirin, ibuprofen, naproxen, or ketoprofen as directed to relieve pain and inflammation. (Acetaminophen relieves pain but has no effect against inflammation; ask your doctor or pharmacist for guidance.)

> **WARNING**
>
> MEDICATIONS
>
> Take the following precautions with medications:
>
> - If you are allergic to aspirin or if you have a history of peptic ulcers, you should not take ibuprofen, naproxen, or ketoprofen; ask your doctor about this.
> - Do not drink alcohol if you are taking aspirin, acetaminophen, ibuprofen, naproxen, or ketoprofen; combining these painkillers with alcohol increases the risk of liver damage or stomach bleeding.
> - If you are pregnant or nursing, talk to your doctor before taking any medication, even one sold over the counter.
> - Never give aspirin to a child under 18 years because the drug is linked to a life-threatening condition called Reye's syndrome in children.

Continued Care Rest your legs for approximately 1 to 3 weeks, depending on the extent of the injury. Use an ice pack on the injury at least once a day for 2 to 4 days after stopping the activity to reduce swelling and inflammation. Use a heating pad thereafter. Heat increases blood circulation in the area, providing vital nutrients to the injury and helping speed recovery. *Do not* apply heat before the swelling has subsided, or swelling in the injured area may increase. Take aspirin, ibuprofen, naproxen, or ketoprofen as directed to reduce the pain and inflammation.

Occasional use of an elastic bandage on the upper leg will help relieve pressure by compressing the quadriceps and hamstring muscles. However, if you have peripheral vascular disease or diabetes, consult your physician first before using an elastic bandage because it can constrict blood circulation. Keep your legs slightly elevated and extended straight out in front of you whenever you can.

Do not engage in the activity that caused the injury until the pain has subsided. Gradually and carefully bend and stretch your leg. Work with a trainer or physical therapist on light exercises that strengthen the hamstring and quadriceps muscles. Use an ice pack to reduce any swelling that may occur. Take aspirin, ibupro-

fen, naproxen, or ketoprofen as directed to relieve pain and inflammation. If the pain continues or if the injury recurs, see your
physician. With proper rest and rehabilitation, a hamstring muscle
pull seldom has any long-term effects.

How to Prevent Recurring Injury Warm up properly. Perform exercises that strengthen the hamstring and quadriceps muscles.

SHIN SPLINT

While not a medical term, "shin splint" denotes the anatomical location of pain that occurs in the front of the lower leg. A shin
splint can be one of several injuries: a tiny tear in a muscle (the
posterior tibial muscle) at the point at which it attaches to the
tibia in the front of the leg, a stress fracture in the bone, or a tiny
tear or inflammation in the thin membrane that covers all the
body's bone surfaces. Anterior compartmental syndrome occurs

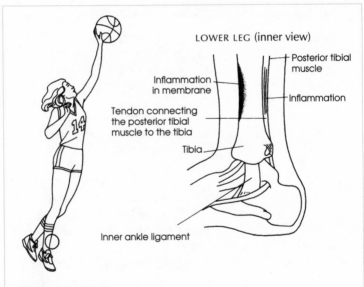

LOWER LEG (inner view)

Posterior tibial muscle

Inflammation in membrane

Inflammation

Tendon connecting the posterior tibial muscle to the tibia

Tibia

Inner ankle ligament

SHIN SPLINT

A shin splint can be one of several injuries including a tiny tear in a muscle, a stress fracture in the lower leg bone, a tiny tear or inflammation in
the membrane that covers the bone surface, or overdevelopment of the
leg muscle. The injury is common in running sports such as basketball.

when exercise increases the size of the muscle in the lower leg, causing the muscle to strain against the surrounding membrane and bone; in serious cases, blood flow to and from the muscles can be restricted.

A tear in the muscle, a stress fracture in the bone, or a tear or inflammation in the membrane covering the bone can all result from overuse, such as during intensive athletic training; from a change in running routine or running surface or shoes; or from participating in sports or vigorous exercise after a period of inactivity. A shin splint can also result from an increase in body weight. Compartmental syndrome results when the leg muscles are overbuilt. Shin splints are common among athletes of all abilities and occur in many sports other than running, including aerobics, baseball, basketball, tennis, rugby, soccer, and walking.

SYMPTOMS

A shin splint causes pain in the lower front portion of the leg. Moving the muscles in the leg worsens the pain.

Immediate Treatment *If the pain in your leg is severe or persistent or if you are unable to walk, see your physician to rule out a stress fracture or anterior compartmental syndrome.*

Stop the activity that is causing the pain. Place an ice pack on the site of the injury intermittently (20 minutes every hour while you're awake) for the first 24 to 48 hours after the injury. Cold treatments help stop internal bleeding and the accumulation of fluids in and around the injured area, thereby decreasing swelling.

Unless your doctor has prescribed another medication, take aspirin, ibuprofen, naproxen, or ketoprofen as directed to relieve pain and inflammation. (Acetaminophen relieves pain but has no effect against inflammation; ask your doctor or pharmacist for guidance.)

SPORTS FIRST AID

> ### WARNING
>
> MEDICATIONS
>
> Take the following precautions with medications:
>
> - If you are allergic to aspirin or if you have a history of peptic ulcers, you should not take ibuprofen, naproxen, or ketoprofen; ask your doctor about this.
> - Do not drink alcohol if you are taking aspirin, acetaminophen, ibuprofen, naproxen, or ketoprofen; combining these painkillers with alcohol increases the risk of liver damage or stomach bleeding.
> - If you are pregnant or nursing, talk to your doctor before taking any medication, even one sold over the counter.
> - Never give aspirin to a child under 18 years because the drug is linked to a life-threatening condition called Reye's syndrome in children.

Continued Care Rest your legs for 3 to 6 weeks. Do not engage in the activity that caused the injury until the pain has subsided. Apply a heating pad to the injury. Heat increases blood circulation in the area, providing vital nutrients to the injury and helping speed recovery. *Do not* apply heat before the swelling has subsided, or swelling in the injured area may increase. Take aspirin, ibuprofen, naproxen, or ketoprofen as directed to reduce the pain and inflammation. Use an ice pack on the area to reduce any swelling that may occur. If the pain continues after you resume activity, see your physician.

With proper treatment and rest, a shin splint seldom has any long-term effects. In serious cases of anterior compartmental syndrome, surgery may be required to cut the membrane (fascia) covering the muscle.

How to Prevent Recurring Injury Work with a trainer or physical therapist to strengthen the surrounding ankle muscles. You may be advised to use shoe inserts that help support the arch and take stress off the lower leg. Resume activity, especially running sports, gradually.

Muscle cramps occur when the muscles tighten up during or after athletic activity, usually when the activity is prolonged, such as during a marathon, an extended tennis match, or a long bicycle ride. Cramps can occur almost anywhere in the body. During athletic activity, cramps can occur in the stomach, legs, feet, arms, neck, or back. Cramps in the legs are very common, especially in the hamstring muscles in the back upper leg, the quadriceps muscles in the front upper leg, and the calf muscles in the back lower leg. Cramps develop when the muscles deplete their supply of oxygen and glycogen, a carbohydrate energy source that is stored

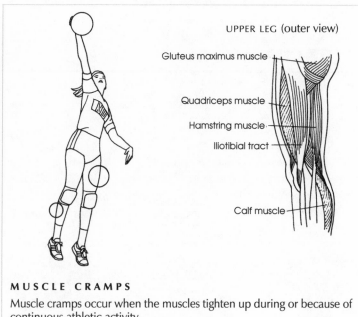

UPPER LEG (outer view)

Gluteus maximus muscle

Quadriceps muscle

Hamstring muscle

Iliotibial tract

Calf muscle

MUSCLE CRAMPS

Muscle cramps occur when the muscles tighten up during or because of continuous athletic activity.

SPORTS FIRST AID

in muscles and in the liver. Cramps can also result from a chemical imbalance in the body, or when the body has insufficient water to help remove waste products.

SYMPTOMS

Muscle cramps can be very painful. Stopping the activity that is causing the cramp can make it worse. However, continuing the activity is often impossible.

Immediate Treatment *Some cramps can be severe. If the cramp is not relieved by massage, or if a heating pad is not available to place on the muscle, see your physician to determine proper treatment.*

Gently stretch out the muscle if possible. Massage it to help work out the cramp. If a heating pad is available, place it on the muscle to help relieve tightness. Continue massaging the muscle until the cramp goes away.

Unless your doctor has prescribed another medication, take aspirin, ibuprofen, naproxen, or ketoprofen as directed to relieve pain and inflammation. (Acetaminophen relieves pain but has no effect against inflammation; ask your doctor or pharmacist for guidance.)

WARNING

MEDICATIONS

Take the following precautions with medications:

- If you are allergic to aspirin or if you have a history of peptic ulcers, you should not take ibuprofen, naproxen, or ketoprofen; ask your doctor about this.
- Do not drink alcohol if you are taking aspirin, acetaminophen, ibuprofen, naproxen, or ketoprofen; combining these painkillers with alcohol increases the risk of liver damage or stomach bleeding.
- If you are pregnant or nursing, talk to your doctor before taking any medication, even one sold over the counter.
- Never give aspirin to a child under 18 years because the drug is linked to a life-threatening condition called Reye's syndrome in children.

Continued Care You can usually resume athletic activity after an attack of cramps. If soreness persists, stop the activity and massage the muscle or use a heating pad to relax it. Take aspirin, ibuprofen, naproxen, or ketoprofen as directed to help relieve the pain and inflammation. See your physician if the cramps occur regularly during exercise or athletic activity. With proper treatment, muscle cramps rarely have any long-term effects.

How to Prevent Recurring Injury Include foods in your diet that are high in potassium and calcium, including bananas, high-fiber cereals or bread, fresh vegetables, milk, yogurt, and cheese. Drink plenty of water before and during extended exercise or athletic activity; water helps the muscles eliminate waste products and helps you avoid dehydration. In some situations, such as engaging in sports during hot weather when the body may be working twice as hard, you might get cramps even when you've taken preventive measures.

The shoulder is a complex ball-and-socket joint consisting of three main bones—the humerus (the upper part of the upper arm bone), the clavicle (the collarbone), and the scapula (or shoulder blade, the largest bone in the chest-shoulder region). The top of the humerus forms the ball in the joint and is attached by ligaments to the shoulder blade. Muscles travel over, under, and around the shoulder joint and provide stability. Tendons connect the muscles to bone. The shoulder allows the hand and arm to move.

SHOULDER DISLOCATION

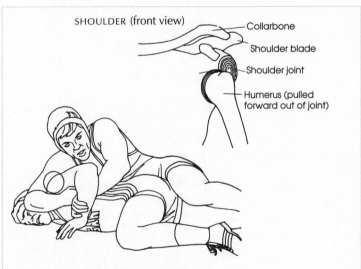

SHOULDER (front view)

— Collarbone

— Shoulder blade

— Shoulder joint

— Humerus (pulled forward out of joint)

SHOULDER DISLOCATION

A dislocated shoulder occurs when the top of the bone in the upper arm (the humerus) is displaced from the joint, usually from a fall or a direct blow to the shoulder.

In most cases of shoulder dislocation, the upper arm bone (humerus) pops out of the joint, usually toward the front. Ligaments, tendons, and other connective tissues are stretched or torn and may injure nerves and blood vessels in the shoulder region, sometimes causing numbness in the hand.

The injury can result from a traumatic event, such as a direct blow to or a fall on the shoulder, or from falling on an outstretched hand or arm. Susceptibility to shoulder dislocation may also be genetic, particularly if the shoulder pops out often or easily. Members of the same family are often affected. In some cases, the shoulder can dislocate during sleep. A shoulder dislocation is common in contact sports, especially football, and sports such as downhill skiing, lacrosse, hockey, volleyball, rugby, and soccer.

SYMPTOMS

A dislocated shoulder causes severe pain the moment the injury occurs. You may experience limited movement in the shoulder area, and swelling and bruising. The shoulder may look abnormal, with a large bump rising up under the skin.

Immediate Treatment *Seek immediate medical treatment at a physician's office or hospital emergency department.*

If possible, on your way to the doctor's office or hospital, apply an ice pack to the shoulder area. Cold treatments help stop internal bleeding and the accumulation of fluids in and around the injured area, thereby decreasing swelling. The shoulder may be put in a sling or wrapped to immobilize the area and aid recovery. (If you have a recurring dislocation, you may be able to pop the shoulder back into place yourself.) Your physician may prescribe a pain-relieving drug, such as codeine with aspirin or acetaminophen. He or she may also recommend a nonsteroidal anti-inflammatory drug such as ibuprofen, naproxen, or ketoprofen to reduce swelling.

> ### WARNING
>
> MEDICATIONS
>
> Take the following precautions with medications:
>
> - If you are allergic to aspirin or if you have a history of peptic ulcers, you should not take ibuprofen, naproxen, or ketoprofen; ask your doctor about this.
> - Do not drink alcohol if you are taking aspirin, acetaminophen, ibuprofen, naproxen, or ketoprofen; combining these painkillers with alcohol increases the risk of liver damage or stomach bleeding.
> - If you are pregnant or nursing, talk to your doctor before taking any medication, even one sold over the counter.
> - Never give aspirin to a child under 18 years because the drug is linked to a life-threatening condition called Reye's syndrome in children.

Continued Care

Do not participate in sports until your shoulder has had time to heal, which may take 3 to 6 weeks, depending on the extent of the injury. With your physician's okay, work with a trainer or physical therapist to strengthen the muscles in the shoulder region. Take aspirin, ibuprofen, naproxen, or ketoprofen as directed to help reduce any pain and inflammation that may occur.

Long-Term Effects With proper healing, the shoulder should regain its full range of motion. In some cases, especially after recurring dislocations, surgery may be recommended to help stabilize the shoulder.

How to Prevent Recurring Injury Avoid situations that could cause another shoulder injury. Wear layers of clothing or padding to help cushion a fall. Use weights and exercises recommended by a trainer or physical therapist to strengthen the muscles in the shoulder region. Muscle-strengthening exercises also help strengthen ligaments and tendons. Use an ice pack to reduce any swelling. After the swelling subsides, use a heating pad.

SHOULDER SEPARATION

A shoulder separation occurs when ligaments that hold the collarbone to the shoulder blade are torn. The collarbone also may be pushed out of alignment.

A shoulder separation usually results from an injury, such as a direct blow to or fall on the shoulder area. It can also result from falling on an outstretched hand or arm. The injury is very common in contact sports, especially football, and sports such as downhill skiing, lacrosse, hockey, volleyball, rugby, and soccer.

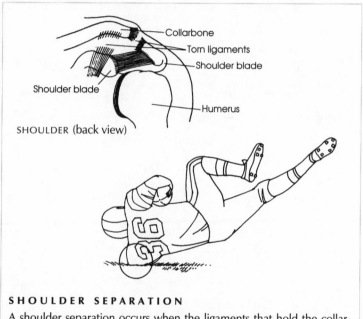

Collarbone
Torn ligaments
Shoulder blade
Shoulder blade
Humerus

SHOULDER (back view)

SHOULDER SEPARATION

A shoulder separation occurs when the ligaments that hold the collarbone to the shoulder blade are torn. The injury can result from a direct blow to or fall on the shoulder.

SYMPTOMS

A shoulder separation causes severe pain the moment the injury occurs. You may experience swelling, bruising, and limited movement in the shoulder area. The shoulder may have an abnormal shape.

Immediate Treatment *This injury always requires professional medical attention. Seek medical treatment at a physician's office or hospital emergency department at once.*

If possible, place an ice pack on the injury right after it occurs. Cold treatments help stop internal bleeding and the accumulation of fluids in and around the injured area, thereby decreasing swelling.

The doctor will put your shoulder in a sling or wrap it to immobilize the area and aid recovery. He or she may prescribe a pain-relieving drug, such as codeine with aspirin or acetaminophen. He or she may also recommend a nonsteroidal anti-inflammatory drug such as ibuprofen, naproxen, or ketoprofen to reduce the pain and swelling.

WARNING

MEDICATIONS

Take the following precautions with medications:

- If you are allergic to aspirin or if you have a history of peptic ulcers, you should not take ibuprofen, naproxen, or ketoprofen; ask your doctor about this.
- Do not drink alcohol if you are taking aspirin, acetaminophen, ibuprofen, naproxen, or ketoprofen; combining these painkillers with alcohol increases the risk of liver damage or stomach bleeding.
- If you are pregnant or nursing, talk to your doctor before taking any medication, even one sold over the counter.
- Never give aspirin to a child under 18 years because the drug is linked to a life-threatening condition called Reye's syndrome in children.

Continued Care Do not participate in sports until the injury has healed, which may take 2 to 10 weeks, depending on the severity. With your physician's okay, work with a trainer or physical therapist to strengthen the muscles in the shoulder region. Take aspirin, ibuprofen, naproxen, or ketoprofen as directed to help reduce the pain and inflammation. See your physician if the pain and swelling reappear or if movement of the shoulder is limited.

Long-Term Effects A shoulder separation usually has no lasting effects. Some people, however, may have pain, stiffness, or limitation of motion in their shoulder. In severe cases, surgery may be necessary; the surgery usually involves removing the outer ½ inch tip of the collarbone.

How to Prevent Recurring Injury Avoid situations that could cause another injury. Wear layers of clothing or padding to help cushion a fall. Use weights and exercises recommended by a trainer or physical therapist to strengthen the muscles in the shoulder region. Muscle-strengthening exercises also help strengthen ligaments and tendons. Once the swelling has subsided, apply a heating pad to aid recovery. Heat increases blood circulation in the area, providing vital nutrients to the injury and helping speed recovery.

SWIMMER'S SHOULDER

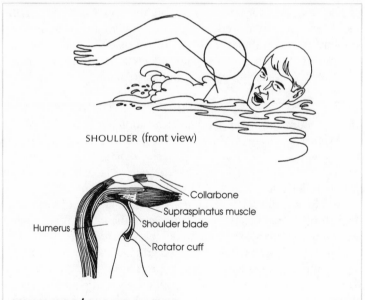

SHOULDER (front view)

Collarbone
Supraspinatus muscle
Shoulder blade
Humerus
Rotator cuff

SWIMMER'S SHOULDER
Swimmer's shoulder is a strain or, sometimes, a tiny tear in the supraspinatus muscle in the shoulder. The injury is usually associated with a repetitive motion over time.

SPORTS FIRST AID

333

Swimmer's shoulder is a strain and, sometimes, a tiny tear, in the supraspinatus muscle on top of the shoulder between the neck and the top of the arm. Swimmer's shoulder can also result from a strain or tear in the rotator cuff, an intertwined unit of muscles and tendons that surrounds and gives stability to the shoulder at the ball-and-socket joint; this injury is called impingement syndrome.

Swimmer's shoulder is usually associated with a repetitive motion over time. It also can occur when a swimmer increases his or her distance or speed, or both, or uses an improper swimming stroke. Other sports that can cause swimmer's shoulder include baseball (pitching), football (passing), tennis (serving), racquetball, volleyball, basketball, golf, sailing, canoeing, kayaking, javelin throwing, shot putting, weight lifting, and rock climbing. Other activities that may cause swimmer's shoulder include those in which the arm is elevated above the head for a prolonged period, such as construction work, painting, plastering, or housework.

SYMPTOMS

Swimmer's shoulder causes pain on the top front part of the shoulder. You may experience pain from lying on your shoulder at night or pain and weakness when you extend the arm forward or upward. You may feel a painful "hitch" in the shoulder and have limited movement in the shoulder joint.

Immediate Treatment *If you cannot extend your arm above your head or move your arm at all ("frozen shoulder"), or if there is a sharp pain and weakness where the arm connects to the trunk, see your physician to determine proper treatment.*

Stop the activity that is causing the pain. Place an ice pack on the shoulder intermittently (20 minutes every hour while you're awake) for the first 24 to 48 hours after the injury. Cold treatments help stop internal bleeding and the accumulation of fluids in and around the injured area, thereby decreasing swelling.

Unless your doctor has prescribed another medication, take aspirin, ibuprofen, naproxen, or ketoprofen as directed to relieve pain and inflammation. (Acetaminophen relieves pain but has no effect against inflammation; ask your doctor or pharmacist for guidance.) For severe inflammation or for a recurring case, your doctor may recommend an injection of a corticosteroid drug such as cortisone.

> ### WARNING
>
> MEDICATIONS
>
> Take the following precautions with medications:
>
> - If you are allergic to aspirin or if you have a history of peptic ulcers, you should not take ibuprofen, naproxen, or ketoprofen; ask your doctor about this.
> - Do not drink alcohol if you are taking aspirin, acetaminophen, ibuprofen, naproxen, or ketoprofen; combining these painkillers with alcohol increases the risk of liver damage or stomach bleeding.
> - If you are pregnant or nursing, talk to your doctor before taking any medication, even one sold over the counter.
> - Never give aspirin to a child under 18 years because the drug is linked to a life-threatening condition called Reye's syndrome in children.

Continued Care Rest your arm for about 4 to 8 weeks. Do not engage in the activity that caused the injury until the pain has subsided. Ease into limited muscle workouts—for example, gradually swing your arm as if throwing a ball, work with light weights, and work with a trainer or physical therapist on light shoulder exercises that use and strengthen the injured muscle. Use an ice pack to help reduce any swelling that may recur, then apply a heating pad to help repair the injury. Take aspirin, ibuprofen, naproxen, or ketoprofen as directed to help reduce pain and inflammation. If the pain continues, is severe, or limits motion in your shoulder, see your physician.

Long-Term Effects With proper treatment and rest, swimmer's shoulder seldom has any long-term effects, although some people experience recurring pain even with preventive measures (see below). In rare cases, surgery may be recommended to remove scar tissue from the rotator cuff area.

SPORTS FIRST AID

How to Prevent Recurring Injury Allow plenty of time for healing. Use weights and exercises recommended by a trainer or physical therapist to strengthen the shoulder muscle. Ask a swimming instructor or baseball or football coach about proper technique. You may need to continue to do these exercises throughout your life to avoid or reduce pain in your shoulder.

MEDICAL CHART

Family Members (Names)	Allergies	Major Medical Problems (DATE)	Medications (DATE)	Tetanus Booster (DATE)	Influenza (DATE)

eumococcal neumonia (DATE)	*Haemophilus influenzae* type b (DATE)	Hepatitis B (DATE)	Polio (DATE)	Diptheria-Tetanus-Pertussis (DPT) (DATE)	Measles-Mumps-Rubella (DATE)	Other Medical Information

INDEX